BOOK 3

TAKE A *Step* WITH *Him*

ADVENTURING WITH GOD INTO FRESH BEGINNINGS

KAREN BROUGH

Written by a very natural girl and a supernatural God

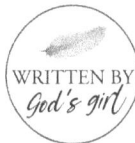

WRITTEN BY
God's girl

SOME REAL PEOPLE'S RESPONSES:

The 3rd book in Karen's raw and honest series that documents her journey from pain and despair to hope and promise is all you could hope it would be. Be encouraged, comforted and inspired as you journey with Karen into a place of fresh beginnings, as you learn to hear God with clarity and trust. As you consistently see Him at work in your life, your relationship with Him will blossom and grow. May this book bless you and inspire you to press in to Him and all that He has for you.

—Julie Jones

This series is an excellent witness of God's truth. Each chapter brings a different insight into the character of God and how to connect with Holy Spirit daily. I have personally been learning how to stay connected to Holy Spirit in all I do, and Karen brings that concept into reality.

I get more excited through each chapter as Christ shines brighter and brighter. Karen provides such keen insights of Holy Spirit and how to best continue forward in cooperation with God in every season of life. It is such a precious journey Karen brings each reader through as we experience glimpses of her life and testimony of who God forever is. What an encouragement!

Oh, that we will all tap into the heart of God moment by moment and share those stories with those around us. Be blessed and encouraged to action as you read this book.

—Sonya Loso

I continue to be amazed at how God is using this book to reveal to me the next steps of my journey with Him. It's as if the curtains of darkness and uncertainty have been pulled back to let the light of God's Word shine through. Each chapter, I get glimpses of the abundant life that God has for me and how I can walk in that abundant life while experiencing the difficulties of life in this world of brokenness. The secret is allowing the Holy Spirit to fill and enable me.

I love how the author so vulnerably shares her own struggles that led to this revelation. In this manner, I realize that this breakthrough is possible for me as well. As I have said before, I can see my life story alongside hers and realize that if God can restore her joy, I can find His joy too.

—Deb Chatley

To the ones who consider themselves
(or at least want to)...

Overcomers...

Battlers...

Warriors...

To the weak and the vulnerable...

God is all that we are not, and in this,
we are never without what we need.

In this, all that we are not, we actually ARE.

God bless you, dearly loved overcomer;
strong, robust warrior of His.

And to my most beloved Father God,

Papa, You have made the darkest moments like the noonday sun.

Life just isn't life without You.

XXXXX

EDITOR

*(The ultimate language artist, accomplished, generous,
and precious new friend from across the oceans)*

Linda Stubblefield | affordablechristianediting.com

PROOFREADING AND EDITING GIFT-STRAIGHT FROM GOD.

Wise, empathetic, intuitive, and Father's heart girl,
Julie Jones, God bless you and yours, chickadee.

GRAPHIC CONCEPT DESIGN

(The intuitive, talented creative heart and developer of dreams)

Abigail Parker | abigail@sponge.com.au

MAP ILLUSTRATOR

*(The courageous, gifted, illustrative visionary
and Holy Spirit led, heart woman of His)*

Stacey Leitch | staceyleitch.com

BOOK COVER DESIGN & FORMATTING

*(The oh so patient, professional, full of integrity,
skilled book creative and design king)*

Steve Kuhn | kuhndesigngroup.com

Contents

LETTER TO THE READER

Precious reader,

If you've reached this final book in the *Be Held By Him* series, I know that you will be seeing, hearing and experiencing God in ways that bless your daily life.

Take heart! There is always more to encounter of God, and what a bizarre and incredible thought it is, that we will never reach the end of this experience!

My encouragement to you is this:

Dive in!

If it's good...

If it reflects His heart...

If it is aligned with Scripture and Jesus' model,

Dive in! Go for it!

What's stopping you from relishing life as fully as you can — in this place you find yourself. You are so much more than your situation, diagnosis or feeling. If any of us have breath, then we have purpose. I hope these simple stories assure you of that truth.

Hindrances or not, God has ways for you to flourish — right now.

And that, beloved reader, is my prayer for you...

That you would flourish with Him.

And on the days where you feel it beyond you, that you'd allow Him to replenish, restore and encourage you. That you'd know He isn't loading more weight upon you, but has plans to lighten those loads and lift those burdens.

Thank you for going on this journey with me.

If you have enjoyed these books, I share many more God stories, encouragement and life-giving hope through karenbrough.com. The journey doesn't stop with this book, there is more to come.

There is more to live and more to celebrate—always more because He is abundantly GOOD.

I look forward to cheering you on and celebrating what He is doing in your life too.

With much love,

Karen
xxxxx

EXPLANATION OF THE MAP

"The Journey" map outlines the various chapters of each book in the *Be Held by Him* series. "The Journey" reveals a story of how God can speak to and interact with us, especially in the hard seasons of life.

I hope you look at the map (especially in hard seasons) and ask God how He wants to speak to you today. Look at the map and see what word/chapter leaps out to your heart…then start there.

God bless you in the valleys and the mountaintops.

I pray the map both encourages and invests hope in your heart.

With God by your side, there is always so much more to look forward to!

Don't give up!

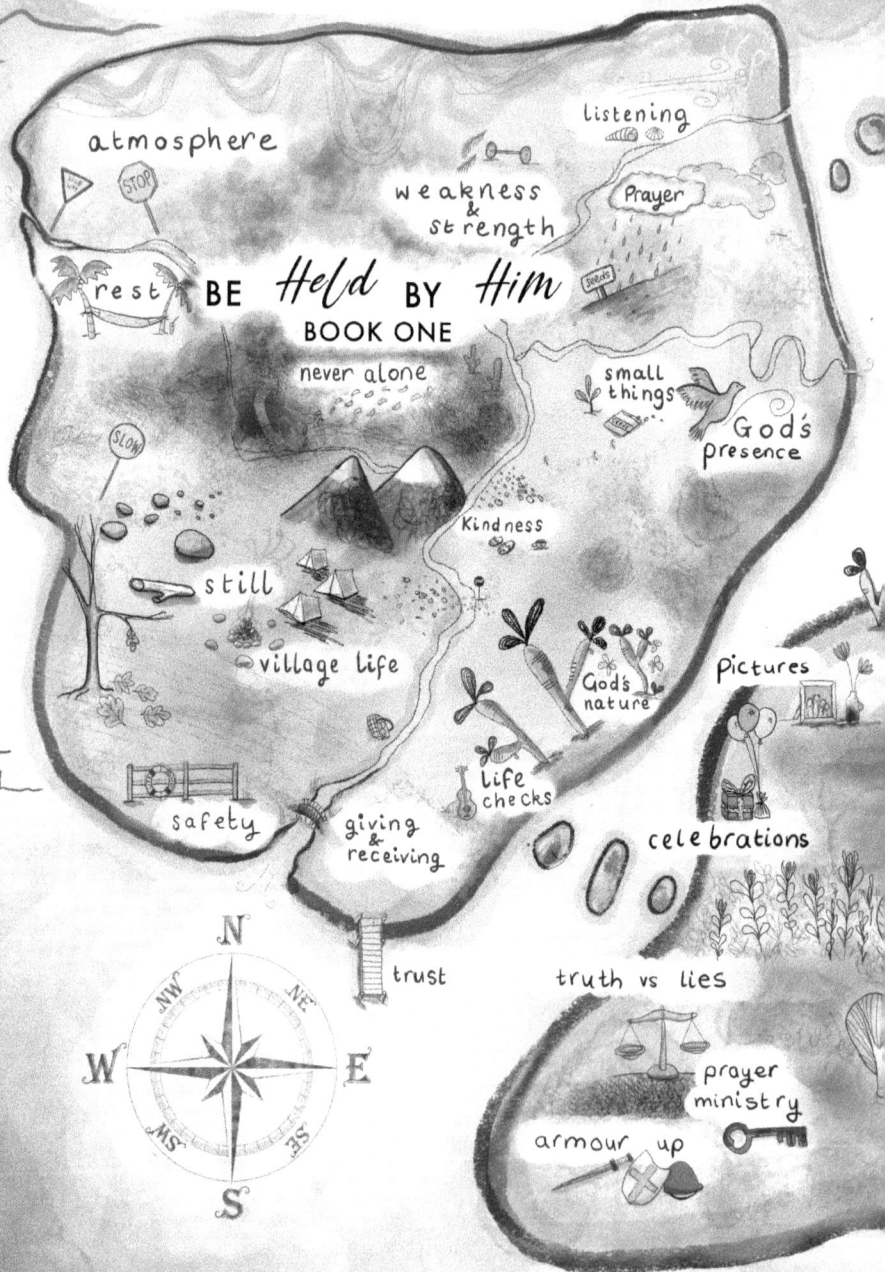

The Journey

atmosphere

listening

weakness & strength

Prayer

STOP

rest

BE *Held* BY *Him*

BOOK ONE

never alone

small things

God's presence

SLOW

Kindness

still

God's nature

village life

pictures

safety

giving & receiving

life checks

celebrations

trust

truth vs lies

N
NW NE
W E
SW SE
S

prayer ministry

armour up

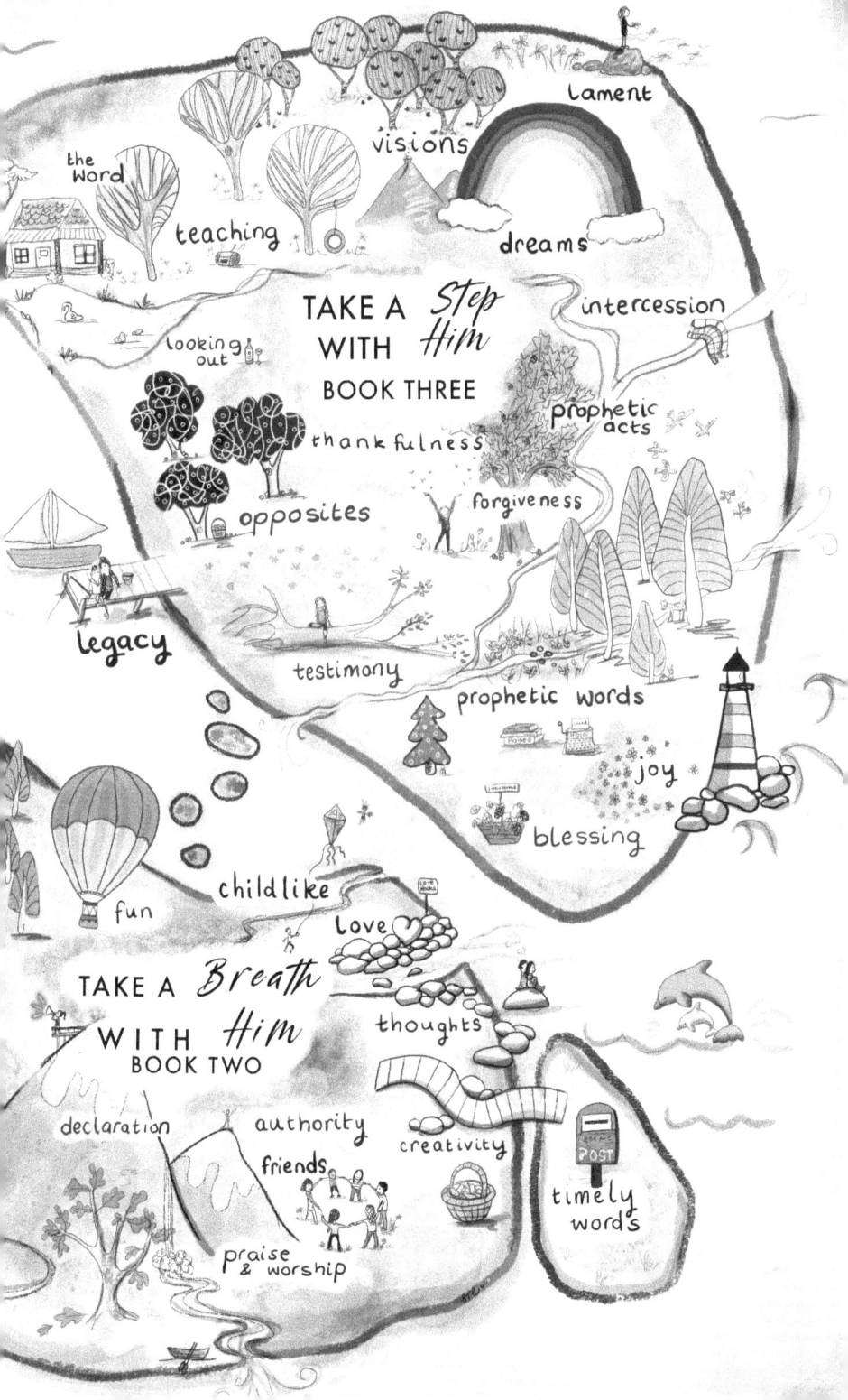

A QUICK PROVISO:

You might notice as you read that I don't use the traditional term "The Holy Spirit." This is a personal choice for me, and by no means do I wish to cause offense to anyone who thinks differently.

Each triune part of God—Father, Jesus, and Holy Spirit—is tangible, alive, and personable, complete, but each connects with me in different ways.

For me to address the Holy Spirit as "The Holy Spirit" would be to hold Him at a distance, and I want Him as near as possible. Please feel free to add "the" if that designation fits with how you communicate with Him.

Bless you, precious one.

XXXXX

A WORD OF WARNING

The following is my personal "beginning" health story that could contain some triggering aspects for those in raw places.

If you are in this place, you may want to consult the contents page for a chapter that speaks directly to your heart.

"Take a Step with Him" is the third book in the "Be Held by Him" series, and it provides the origin story, offering context for readers who are new to the series, or who haven't read "Be Held by Him" or "Take a Breath with Him."

Where It All Began

L ying on the bed, unable to move my limbs, head, and body, my heart wept. *Am I dying? Is this IT? What about my hubby Craig and the kids?* Thoughts were racing in and out, endeavouring to find a place to land, to find order and explanation…but at that moment, there was none to find.

The constant headache of the past six weeks hadn't slowed me. I pushed through, taking paracetamol to ease the knifelike pangs to no avail. I pushed on, meeting the commitments, the pressures of being a wife, a mum, a business partner, a teacher, the various voluntary committees, responsibilities, and relationships—everything cried out for more—of me. That small voice within screamed for me to slow down, but in my mind, I simply had no time…

No time to stop…

No time to consider and ask what was causing the unfamiliar symptom…

No time to cull the calendar craziness…

No time to be still…

No time…

No time…

No time…

It'll have to wait became a common thought during this time, prioritizing everyone else but myself. After all, sacrificing myself for others is what…real service is about, isn't it? I was a servant-hearted wife of one, the mother of three, and now I couldn't do a thing.

My body had sent out the warning signs—the unheeded flashing red lights trying their best to let me know things weren't right. I hadn't listened, and now, I'd pushed beyond my body's limits. Layer upon layer of the past year's stresses flooded to mind as I lay there, waiting for the ambulance to arrive.

MY BODY HAD ENDURED ENOUGH! I NOW HAD NO CHOICE; MY BODY WOULD TAKE WHAT IT NEEDED — WITH OR WITHOUT MY PERMISSION.

Pale, exhausted, unable to lift a single finger, I was now at the whim of life and circumstances. My body had endured enough! I now had no choice; my body would take what it needed—with or without my permission.

Lying there, so filled with weakness that nothing would function as I willed it to, fear expanded within.

Terror seized my distress, and they embraced. As the seconds passed, new symptoms appeared, and I felt as though life was leaving me. My eyes closed, and I tried desperately to come to peace with what I was leaving behind.

My family, oh, my precious family—Craig, my children.

Just moments before, in our first extended family dinner in months, we had been busy catching up around the dinner table. Everyone was able to be present. What a delight! So good to be back at the family home.

Squeals of joy came from our kids and their cousins as they played happily in the background. Mum and Dad were in the kitchen cleaning up, and my sister and I bantered back and forth across the table, having some good hearty laughs. These times were precious.

My family was so dear to me. Together is the place I wanted to be all the time. These nights were a balm for my soul.

Then, in a split second, everything changed.

My eyes moved of their own accord, as if some mysterious fingers were pulling the muscles behind them. My neck became sore, stiff, and the slight headache intensified.

My body felt the waves of nausea and fatigue HIT, and boy, did it hit! Any energy I had dissipated and withdrew, heading who knows where. Beginning with my extremities, I felt as if my blood was retreating. My hands weakened, and my arms fell limply to each side of my body. My head joined the procession and dropped upon my shoulder. The weightiness of it propelled my immobilized body to the right—where Craig sat.

"Catch me, honey," I barely breathed out as my entire body fell on his lap.

Apart from the sheer physical exhaustion and my brain's feeling as though it was splitting in two, I don't remember much of the following minutes. My listless, unresponsive form was carried to my parents' bedroom nearby, and an ambulance was called.

Time stood still, and I couldn't comprehend much of what anyone was saying. Every cell in my body felt weighty—sleepy, as if the energy had been sucked out of every molecule. They demanded rest, and rest they did.

The medical staff arrived, and the family tension was relieved on some level for a moment. The cavalry had arrived, and now they could "fix" Karen.

The paramedics took my vitals and eventually surmised that I was "…just a tired mum" as they offered to transport me to the hospital, while articulating that they wouldn't do much for me there. Confusion…upset…shock remained.

Ever so slightly, a minuscule amount of strength found its way to my extremities, and my limbs began to be able to move once again. They felt weighty and slow-moving—like I was on heavy medication or in recovery from surgery. But the exhaustion remained.

I remember Craig asking what I wanted to do. I remember not wanting to or being able to decide. My brain had ceased to be able to think coherently. The decision was made not to go to the hospital, and as the ambulance officers left, the hope of help seemed to depart with them.

Inside, my questions mounted: *how could they leave me here like this? What is going to happen?*

Soon after, we headed home as if nothing had happened.

The only thing was something HAD happened and was indeed happening. My body had never felt such fatigue before. I felt as if I'd been hit by a Mack truck or run a 100km marathon in a moment. Every part of me ached and screamed, "I'm so weary!"

I remained silent. No one spoke on the way home. The fear was palpable, and no one knew what to say. Ours was the quietest car trip our family had ever had.

The sounds of the tires on the road hurt my head; the glare of the streetlights stung my eyes. Sitting upright was a challenge, as my head felt like a bowling ball. As we rattled along, my head leaned against the cold passenger window with every bump, every knock, every turn felt and intensified. This was the longest car trip I'd ever had.

I plopped into bed, desperate for sleep. My eyelids closed as a signal for the soon-to-come sleep to come that successfully evaded me much of that night.

Fearful thoughts raced around and persisted for hours as the shock and trauma of what had occurred replayed inside my mind. A new seed of affliction and fear had been planted that night and would endeavour to wreak havoc in our lives for many months and years to come.

The next morning, I woke, meaning I must've slept, but I felt no benefit, no refreshment or renewed energy. My eyelids were heavy; my brain matter felt as if it was crystallizing inside like crackling ice as the temperature warms. So too was my head and its sensitivity to everything. The whole-body weakness persisted, and I struggled to stand, to talk, or to walk upright.

A barrage of thoughts tried to rattle my weary frame. *You have a brain tumor. You're going to die a slow, painful death. Your family will see it and be powerless. It'll be painful for them too. It's going to get worse…* Many more painful thoughts permeated my mind.

I was in the space of sheer terror; my pupils dilated almost wholly, and my snowlike complexion showed things were not as they should be. Something was desperately wrong, and I was without solutions. I felt a small and insignificant voice in a body that refused to obey my commands anymore.

A NEW SEED OF AFFLICTION AND FEAR HAD BEEN PLANTED THAT NIGHT AND WOULD ENDEAVOUR TO WREAK HAVOC IN OUR LIVES FOR MANY MONTHS AND YEARS TO COME.

I don't remember thinking of or speaking to God much during this time; I allowed fear to reign mostly in this space.

All I could squeak out in a moment of reprieve was a single word: "Help!"

He heard my cry, and help came.

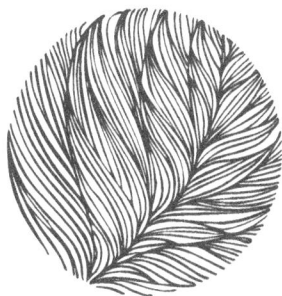

Chapter One

TESTIMONY

And we know that God causes all things to work together for good to those who love God, to those who are called according to His purpose.

ROMANS 8:28 NLT

But because the LORD loves you, and because He would keep the oath which He swore to your fathers, the LORD has brought you out with a mighty hand, and redeemed you from the house of bondage, from the hand of Pharaoh king of Egypt.

DEUTERONOMY 7:8 NKJV

The car sped along the freeway, as trees, houses, and grassland passed by.

Heading home from our regular chiropractic adjustment, my body not unlike the car, hummed.

It felt great to have had an adjustment, but unfortunately, the procedure had left my nervous system buzzing.

My mind wandered and zoned out a little.

A picture unfolded in my mind's eye. I was in front of a large crowd, sharing my life story.

That image, being in front of a large group, that is the thing of nightmares.

Groan. *Oh no, I hate public speaking!*

My heart raced, and palms became sweaty at the thought.

Who am I to say no if God wants it?

The trees and power lines zipped by, one after the other.

The radio played several songs, but I wasn't paying attention.

Maybe it would be okay?

I do love telling God stories, and what He has done. Hmmmm…

Peace.

The heart palpitations and anxiety settled.

HOW IS LIFE
MEASURED? BY
PAINS? OR JOYS?

If You want it, Lord, I'd do it…even if I find it hard. I'd be happy to share what You've done!

My family chattered away in the background, enjoying the drive home.

As we passed the farmlets on both sides, the picture and intricacies of speaking to a group grew in my thoughts.

What would I say?

What would I include, and what would I omit? What is my story?

The years of trouble, trauma, and affliction began listing off in my mind. Pages, books of life-changing events, attacks, strife, and as I took stock of the years one by one, I found myself unable to know how far back to go.

My heart was saddened by the plethora of lowlight events of my life.

Where did it all begin?

How is life measured? By pains? Or joys?

What if my lows outweigh the highs?

The corners of my mouth sank as I blankly stared off into the distance.

My story stinks, Lord. Why would I want to share it? It would depress people—not uplift them. And that is opposite of who I am.

The original picture panned out, revealing more of what I hadn't seen in the first place.

As I shared my story, I saw some people felt sorry for me; some lapped up the life gossip; others were in tears; and some found themselves triggered as I shared something that reflected their own experience.

In my mind, most of the speaking time was spent covering the heavy main events.

My body began to ping and pang like lightening during an electrical storm-flash, bang, baz-ing!

This is the opposite of what I want people to experience or walk away with. How do I tell my story authentically, Lord?

I don't want to sugar-coat the hard events. How do I honour You when so many painful things have happened? How do I share without it seeming like You were completely absent?

Time passed as I grappled with this problem of how to express the good God things without getting stuck in the detail of the awful.

The car rumbled along.

I noted a favourite, familiar tree; my eyes welcomed the sweet distraction. It had always piqued my curiosity, with its woven grey bark and ninety-degree angle.

I love that tree.

All the other trees around it stood, tall, straight and upright. Their branches stretched symmetrically, as "all good trees should." The twisted tree had at some point fallen sideways, and there it remained.

TESTIMONY

Its roots were planted deeply in the soil, its trunk as thick as a large serving platter. It was branchless; these had been strategically pruned. This living tree now formed a kind of bench seat.

To others, it might've seemed out of place and broken, but to me... to me, it was an image of hope.

I can relate to this tree.

This tree is me.

Its brokenness had been repurposed and upgraded. The tree now served the landowners faithfully as a place to take a load off and rest for a while.

Yes, it isn't like the others, but neither was I.

My mind stilled and became peaceful, happily taking in the rolling green hills and expansive paddocks filled with livestock.

Ask Me what *My* story of your life is, beloved.

The moment I heard this, my spirit quickened.

What is His story of my life? His story?

He has a story of me?

LIFE FILLED MY CORE AS I PONDERED... GOD'S TESTIMONY OF MY LIFE.

A smile found its way to my lips as I thought upon the possibility of His having a story of me. I considered the depth of what He had just expressed to me.

God's story of my life?

God's story of my life...

God's story of my life!

The same vision replayed except this time I watched as God's version of my story played out. Adventure, excitement, and hope bubbled up as I shared with the group His version of my story.

In every single bad event, trouble, and trauma, He was at work in it all. I saw Him bringing redemption at every turn…

Providing the right people at exactly the right moment,

Protecting me from even worse things that the enemy had planned,

Becoming the very thing I needed — whatever came, my Comforter, Encourager, Healer, Peace and my Friend.

He brought them all and more…

My story became one of God's hand at work, rather than skirmishes and strife — His reframed, upgraded view became mine in an instant.

As a result, I began making a different list: His testimony of my story.

It reads so differently, Lord.

Life filled my core as I pondered…God's testimony of my life.

I'd been focusing on the story of *my* life — my poorly filtered, broken version was a snippet of what had happened. Mine was a version of the truth — but not a whole one.

As we motored along, God revealing His fully redemptive story of my life.

One tear, then another and another trickled down my cheeks, as I experienced His version of my life.

My heart swelled with joy, my mind filling with good thoughts, my body encountered God's version in surround sound and sensory delight.

Sitting there, surrounded by my family—our kids playing in the backseat. Craig, in the driver's seat beside me, turned his head, and noticing my wet cheeks, he asked, "You okay, honey? What's going on?"

In a completely different mindset now, one of hope and anticipation. I looked back at Craig and began sharing all that God had shared. With a single thought, He had turned everything right side up.

How much more can He do with a life that looks through His vision?

What had happened in this car trip proved to be life-changing. The hardships of the past were being reframed by Him and further healing came along with it.

to strengthen those *crushed by despair* who mourn in Zion —
to give them a beautiful bouquet in the place of ashes,
the oil of bliss instead of tears,
and the mantle of joyous praise
instead of the spirit of heaviness.
Because of this, they will be known as
Mighty Oaks of Righteousness,
planted by Yahweh as a *living* display of his glory.

ISAIAH 61:3 TPT

In the past he permitted all the nations to go their own ways, but he never left them without evidence of himself and his goodness. For instance, he sends you rain and good crops and gives you food and joyful hearts.

ACTS 14:16-17 NLT

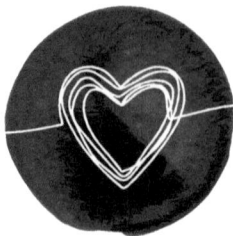

— Father's Heart —

I know that you've endured so much,
My child, but I was with you.

I know you have had some difficult beginnings and find
yourself in challenging circumstances. My heart is grieved by
the injustices and disappointments you have experienced.

All you've experienced will not be wasted.

I have travelled this road with you and comforted
you during it, knowing a time would come where
the things you have had to endure would accomplish
My good purposes. Yes, even from within it.

I will bring you up out of this place with My mighty hand!

None of these are wasted in Me. Your story and your experiences
will be used powerfully and mightily in My name.

I want to redeem the very things that have held you
back, pulled you down or sought to steal your future.

I have the power, ability, and desire to do
this for you because I love you.

You are My child whom I love.

Trust Me, My precious child. Trust Me with your past, your present, and your future. Trust Me with the ups and downs. Trust Me in the bad news, the life shocks and troubles — I am ever-present, ready to partner with you and bring you all that you need at any moment.

My testimony of your life is very different to how it feels in the moment.

When you find yourself reflecting upon the challenges or past struggles...Stop!

Take a moment. Breathe with Me.

Ask Me how I see the thing that captivates your thoughts.

Let Me take your hand, helping you to take the next step forward. It won't always be comfortable, but I do promise you that I will be with you. You won't ever be alone.

I promise you that these things that were sent to take your eyes off Me will strengthen our relationship...if you'll let Me in.

Those hard things will accomplish great things through Me.

My heart loves to beat to the tune of Redeemer, Redeemer, Redeemer — this is exactly Who I am. And it is exactly what I love to do for you, beloved.

Let Me share with you how I've been by your side all along. Let Me reveal to you how your story is entwined with Mine.

Our stories together make for redemptive, sweet, and joyous living.

Come, delight of My heart, let's walk a while together. I will show you marvellous things that will lighten your load and uplift your heart.

TESTIMONY

Since we believe human testimony, surely we can
believe the greater testimony that comes from
God. And God has testified about His Son.

I JOHN 5:9 NLT

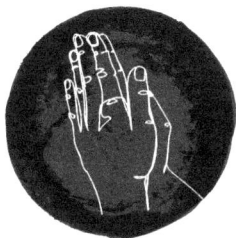

— *Prayer* —

Redemptive God, One Who has the truth-filled vision of my life,

It's a gift, to see things through Your vision.

*I recognize that I am only able to experience life one
dimensionally at times, but You…You see all, wholly complete.*

*Let my heart, mind, and mouth, know, feel, see, speak
and experience Your good testimony of my life.*

*Thank You for being there before I was born. I trust
You have been guiding and loving me all along.*

*Thank You for Your precious Son Jesus and all that He
accomplished through His death and resurrection for me.*

Thank You for the gifts of relationship and adoption by You, Father.

*I appreciate that You turn bad for good, terrifying for peaceful,
the ashes to become beautiful memory stones of my life.*

I love You.

*I love Your ways. Please continue to reveal more
of Your life-giving, hope-filled sight.*

In the redemptive, grace-filled, loving name of Jesus.

Amen.

XXXXX

TESTIMONY

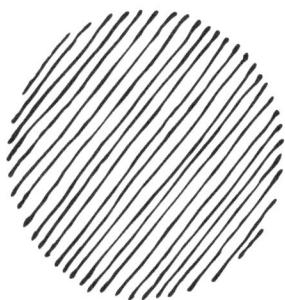

Chapter Two

FORGIVENESS

Therefore there is now no condemnation at
all for those who are in Christ Jesus.

ROMANS 8:1 NKJV

Do not judge [others self-righteously], and you will not be judged; do not condemn [others when you are guilty and unrepentant], and you will not be condemned [for your hypocrisy]; pardon [others when they truly repent and change], and you will be pardoned [when you truly repent and change].

LUKE 6:37 AMP

Sitting in my friend Julie's lounge room, we talked about life and the current challenges regarding my healing.

"If only I'd listened to my body at the beginning, Jules. I'd had that headache for six weeks-why didn't I do something about it?

Why didn't I stop?

Why didn't I go to the doctors and get things checked out?

Why didn't I slow down?

I just kept going. I kept pushing through.

Why?"

I'd raced about for so long in stress mode, unable to deal with any of it. Taking paracetamol for weeks, without stopping long enough to realise it wasn't helping…

Like a shaken can of soda, I burst into tears — a precious release of energy from within.

Thank You, God, for this safe place with Julie to share.

We began to pray about it all, and I blurted out a plethora of self-judgments regarding my lack of self-care.

Julie gently asked, "Karen, have you been able to forgive yourself?"

My head began inadvertently shaking from side to side.

Forgive myself?

Forgive myself...what does that even mean?

I've forgiven doctors and medical practitioners. I'd forgiven those who had spoken harmful words and done damaging things.

But forgive myself...hmmm.

Following a prompt from God, I'd spent months strategically asking God to highlight people I needed to forgive.

I desired to forgive and hated holding onto conflict or offense. Some days new levels, fresh aspects of unforgiveness weighed heavily upon my body systems; it was tangible—I'd discovered. Forgiveness was required for my health to be restored. So, forgive I did!

I knew unforgiveness could hold back healing from me. I'd experienced it. I'd also experienced the freedom that came when forgiveness was given—when God exchanged the pain for His peace about a person or situation.

But never in my wildest dreams had I considered the idea of forgiving myself.

Wasn't that Jesus' job? Why do I need to forgive myself? How can I forgive myself?

You forgive others readily, My daughter.

You ask for forgiveness and allow Me to forgive you.

But you struggle to give yourself that same forgiveness which others receive from you.

*Woah…*humbled…*true.*

My heart swirled with all He had said-that was until I remembered Julie was in the room and realised I'd better share what had been happening.

"What does 'forgive myself' mean, Jules?"

"Well, it means not holding the past and its decisions against yourself. It's about giving yourself as much compassion and kindness as you give to others…and that Jesus gives to you."

As Julie said those words about giving compassion to others, the tears began to flow fresh. She handed me the box of tissues, and we took some time.

No rush, no pressure — just being.

I breathed out a fresh sigh as God unravelled this mess in my heart.

I find it so much easier to be kind to others than myself, Lord.

Are others more valuable than you, My child?

I say No!

You are more precious to Me than you'll ever know.

I love your heart. I love that you seek peace with others. It's time to receive My inner peace for yourself.

More tears.

"Do you feel like this might be something you want to do today, Karen?" Julie gently asked.

As had happened many, many times before, God had put His finger on the pulse of what was needed and spoken powerfully through a gentle prompt from Julie. What a gift!

As I'd done so many times for others, I prayed to God through a process of forgiveness, except this time, it wasn't for others.

It was for me.

The air in the room was stilled, quiet…holy.

God's presence was thick, protective and tangible, like a warm winter blanket covering my raw.

"Thank You, God, for bringing this to my attention.

Thank You for understanding my heart and wanting something better for me.

I'm sorry for holding onto unforgiveness. I think at my core, I believed I deserved punishment for my mistakes. I thought that by feeling it, it would mean I wouldn't make the same mistakes. I thought a lot of things, Father, but I was wrong. With Your help, today, I forgive myself for all of it."

THE AIR IN THE ROOM WAS STILLED, QUIET…HOLY.

I envisioned Jesus holding a bucket and handed Him each of the emotions and judgments, labelling whatever God brought to my mind. I watched Jesus place them in the bucket.

"Please forgive me, Lord, for holding onto it.

I give You the fear, shame, guilt, self-condemnation, judgment, and I choose to release it all to You, Jesus."

Peace.

"Jesus, can You get rid of all that I've given You, please?"

I watched in my mind's eye how He showed me the inside of the bucket and the burnt contents that had become cinders. The ashen particles then disappeared altogether.

Jesus just smiled His reassuring, loving smile. He showed me the clean, empty bucket — ready for the next load of anything I wanted to give Him in the future.

Physically lighter.

I felt freer than I had in years, and a wide grin made its way across my mouth.

> AS I SAT THERE, IT WAS AS IF LARGE, FAT DROPS OF PEACE FELL FROM THE CEILING!

Thank You, Jesus.

The precious silence was a delight. The sense of deep satisfaction which landed within was the kind that comes after accomplishing something significant.

As I sat there with my eyes closed, nestling back into the couch cushions, enjoying the sweet space, Julie broke the silence.

"Holy Spirit, would You reveal to Karen what You want to give her in exchange for all she's let go of today?"

As I sat there, it was as if large, fat drops of peace fell from the ceiling!

The sensation of having each one land on my face, one by one — an unexpected surprise and blessing to my weary body. As they landed, each expanded, spreading and joining with one next to it. I never knew God rained on people who were inside, but His "rain" was a welcome encounter.

A new level of peace was present, a fresh level of freedom.

FORGIVENESS

Sitting there, for who knows how long, my soul was drenched in His peace.

The memory and rawness I had once felt about who I was before the collapse was no longer an open wound, but one that had been cleansed, tended to and gently touched by His healing hand.

I looked at Karen of the past. That woman back there was working so hard to live up to the pace of life. So heavy with all that she expected of herself. In truth, she was working overtime at simply surviving.

I no longer judged her…but had compassion for her and blessed her.

I no longer felt anger and bitterness towards her and her failure to listen to the warning signs; Instead, I felt like hugging her and telling her it was going to be okay. I took a moment to thank her and bless her, letting the Karen of old know the pressure is off and she can rest.

God had indeed done a mighty work with one simple line: "Have you considered forgiving yourself?"

I walked in one woman and walked out a completely different one — a freer, happier, and more peaceful one. Thank You, Lord!

Instead, be kind to each other, tenderhearted, forgiving one another, just as God through Christ has forgiven you.

EPHESIANS 4:31-32 NLT

Repent therefore and be converted, that your sins may be blotted out, so that times of refreshing may come from the presence of the Lord, and that He may send Jesus Christ, who was preached to you before, whom heaven must receive until the times of restoration of all things, which God has spoken by the mouth of all His holy prophets since the world began.

ACTS 3:19-20 NKJV

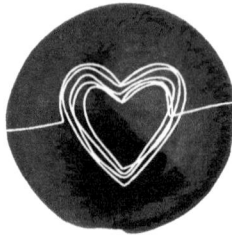

— Father's Heart —

*I have come that you might have life and life to the
full. Sin, poor choices, and unhealthy mindsets are
the world's currency; My currency is higher and
lives far above these things. Why live as a pauper
in the gutter when you are destined for royalty!*

Time to release the old to make way for the new.

*My precious child, I have forgiven you freely. I have
released you from those heavy chains of burden. You
no longer have to live under the weight of them.*

*You're aware of My higher way. You've come to Me,
asking for forgiveness which I've given to you freely.*

Why, then do you hold things against yourself?

*My precious Son died for those things, so
you didn't have to live under them.*

*Why do you take back those things from which I
have freed you? Is it because you want to feel the
pain…as if you deserve to remain in judgment?*

*That is not Me Who says these things to you. I
judge you no more. I've forgiven you wholly.*

*You've turned from your ways, and yet you sometimes choose
to remember the mistakes you've made and relive them.*

*If you are willing, let Jesus be Jesus. You don't need to
take His place in carrying sin or making payment.*

As I forgive you, then surely you can forgive yourself also.

Let go of all that Jesus forgave you for and has now released.

*Let go of your right to hold something
against yourself My beloved.*

Stop punishing yourself for things I don't even remember.

*Release the things that are holding you back. I
have something good for you in exchange.*

*Know that Jesus died so you don't have to hold onto
mistakes of your past. By holding onto them, they
impact the present and can steal from your future.*

*It's time — time to give yourself the compassion
and mercy that Jesus has given you…and
that you willingly often give to others.*

*Be kind to yourself as you are kind to
others and as Jesus is kind to you.*

*Throw off the former ways to dance freely into fresh
beginnings. Step into wide-open spaces where you've been
forgiven, you forgive others, and where you forgive yourself.*

*Get rid of all bitterness, rage, anger, harsh words, and
slander, as well as all types of evil behaviour.*

FORGIVENESS

Tolerate the weaknesses of those in the family of faith,
forgiving one another in the same way you have been graciously
forgiven by Jesus Christ. If you find fault with someone,
release this same gift of forgiveness to them. For love is
supreme and must flow through each of these virtues. Love
becomes the mark of true maturity. Let your heart be always
guided by the peace of the Anointed One, who called you to
peace as part of his one body. And always be thankful.

COLOSSIANS 3:13-15 TPT

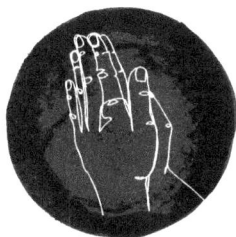

— Prayer —

Father, full of grace, mercy, love and compassion, thank You!

*Thank You for all that You are and all
that You've created me to be.*

*I love that You have higher, better ways of
lifting me from my current place.*

Thank You for forgiveness.

*I love that forgiveness is freeing. Forgiving
others, being forgiven, and even forgiving myself…
thank You that it's all possible with You.*

*Thank You for Your wisdom in knowing what and when to
forgive; please let my heart discern Your promptings well.*

Teach me how to release offense and forgive quickly.

*Prompt my heart to come to You often and keep
short accounts with You and others, Lord.*

Thank You for Your creative solutions and freedom.

Thank You, Jesus, for making it all possible.

In the tender, grace filled name of Jesus,

Amen.

XXXXX

FORGIVENESS

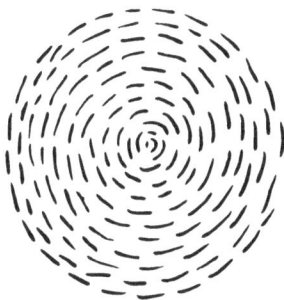

Chapter Three

OPPOSITE

That's why I take pleasure in my weaknesses, and in the insults, hardships, persecutions, and troubles that I suffer for Christ. For when I am weak, then I am strong.

2 CORINTHIANS 12:10 NLT

He does not punish us for all our sins; he does not deal harshly with us, as we deserve. For his unfailing love toward those who fear him is as great as the height of the heavens above the earth.

PSALM 103:10-11 NLT

Walking with purpose, I headed along the front of the strip of shops near the kinder.

It had been a frustrating and upsetting year.

Thank heavens it's November; we're almost done…and I don't ever have to see her again.

She'd done all she could to put wedges between the parents, create conflict, manipulate, and control at every turn.

Loving people who are like this is impossible, Lord!

No thriving this year — just surviving.

Passing by the bakery, the smell of freshly baked bread filled my nostrils.

These are the days I wish I wasn't gluten intolerant. I want to walk into that bakery, order a hot pie with sauce, and an apple cake with pink icing. Some sugar…now, that'd be nice.

LOVING PEOPLE
WHO ARE
LIKE THIS IS
IMPOSSIBLE,
LORD!

My mouth watered at the thought.

A few more shops passed by.

Newsagent, chemist, and bottle shop.

Bottle shop.

Go inside.

What for? I don't drink.

Go inside. Buy her a *really* nice bottle of wine.

I laughed at the thought.

Imagine me going inside. I wouldn't have a clue what I was doing.

Dawdling past the bottle shop, I weighed up how important the prompt was.

I stalled out the front, rummaging around in my bag, as I delayed the inevitable.

I considered bargaining with God.

What if I just got her a gift at Christmastime? It wouldn't seem so weird then.

Now's the time.

Ugh…but I don't really want to. She scares me.

As memories of the intentional angst she had seemed to release — intense — mucked with my mind and heart, I endeavoured to make sense of why someone would behave in this way. She had intimidated and manipulated others as well as me, and truly, I just wanted the year to end, so I didn't have to see her ever again.

Bless her. Make it a really good bottle of wine.

I laughed nervously, as I posted a letter nearby, slowing the process.

I still had half an hour before kinder pickup. Plenty of time to select something and write a card.

Ugh…this is the last thing I want to do.

You're asking me to go into a place I don't know, look like a fool, buy a bottle of wine for someone who considers me an enemy. Surely, I can't be hearing You right…can I, Lord?

Bless those who curse you.

I am smoothing the waves.

In my mind's eye, I saw pictures flash up.

She was sitting at her desk late into the night planning, organising and fundraising for the kindergarten. I felt her stress as she pushed herself to do her role well. She strived and strained. She made no friends by her striving. By being this way, her desire to control outweighed her desire for relational harmony and connection with others. She missed out on so much. I also saw all that her work behind the scenes had brought to benefit the children.

She'd neglected her husband and family. She'd had no holiday break, no vacation that I knew of.

I felt like this might've been a common occurrence for her.

Compassion filled my heart as I considered her life.

As compassion grew, so did a weird and wonderful thing.

Love.

That's strange. A woman who I had once felt so guarded around, I now feel love for.

This is so much better, Lord.

OPPOSITE

I saw all that she'd done and felt appreciative.

Her sacrifice was benefitting the kids.

Yes, she'd been horrible and made the committee and the community a toxic environment, but what if God wanted to infiltrate it?

What if He has plans to do something magnificent?

What if my decision not to follow through with this small request from Him would impact that plan?

Okay, Lord, I'll go.

I zipped up my handbag, made an about-face and headed into the first bottle shop of my life.

The man behind the counter asked in a friendly manner, "Can I help you today?"

I must've looked like a fish out of water as the rows of choices melded into one another.

"What do you recommend as a really good bottle of wine?"

"How much do you want to spend?"

"I've no idea. How much is a really good bottle of wine?"

He laughed and selected a red wine. "This is popular as a gift." The label looked snazzy, and the base of the bottle was deep. A new thing I'd learnt from my new bottle-shop friend.

Relief filled my mind at not having to navigate this by myself.

He wrapped it in a paper bag, I paid him and headed off to grab a card.

Time was ticking by, and I made it to the front gate, just as the children were finishing.

I saw her blonde, bobbed hair swishing about as she made her way through the sea of children.

As I looked at her, I no longer felt like I was at war. All I felt was love for this former bully.

I navigated the way through the sea of giggling, tired ones, eventually finding my target.

> WHAT IF HE HAS PLANS TO DO SOMETHING MAGNIFICENT?

A huge smile spread across my face as I waved to get her attention.

She looked confused, worried and then the stern, regularly pursed lips, "I'm-going-to-tear-shreds-off-you" look settled on her face.

I continued to smile, telling her how much I appreciated all that she'd done.

Unfazed by her battle face, I pressed on.

"I really just wanted to give you a small token to say thank you. The kids are so blessed with the new equipment. They are so happy. We appreciate all that you do. Thank you so much, darlin."

She was floored.

As I handed her the wine and card, her jaw dropped to the ground.

Her cheeks reddened. She looked toward the ground.

Shame.

I thanked her again, cheering her heart and encouraging her.

God had so much to pour into her, and being His bearer of it felt great.

Her face warmed and softened right before my eyes.

OPPOSITE

"Th...tha..thank you, Karen." Obviously affirmed and moved by it all.

"Now go home, run a bath, and pour yourself a glass, you've earned it," I gently suggested.

Her eyes glistened with delight, and she laughed at the thought, releasing a huge sigh.

HER FACE WARMED AND SOFTENED RIGHT BEFORE MY EYES.

Was she tearing up?

I didn't stay long enough to check.

Taking Hannah's hand, we headed to the car. My spirit leapt at what He had just done.

The following last weeks of Kinder were a delight; this new woman was more herself than I'd seen all year. And all of us benefited. No more knifing or nastiness—only a spirit of celebration.

Oh, You are such a redeeming God. Thank You for the prompt. Thank You that activating the opposite of what I feel can often bring breakthrough.

Thank You for teaching me that You are always at work and desire to soften hearts all over...including mine.

When a man's ways are pleasing to the LORD, he
makes even his enemies live at peace with him.

PROVERBS 16:7 NASB 1995

The Spirit of the Sovereign LORD is on me,
because the LORD has anointed me
to proclaim good news to the poor.
He has sent me to bind up the brokenhearted,
to proclaim freedom for the captives
and release from darkness for the prisoners,
to proclaim the year of the LORD's favour
and the day of vengeance of our God,
to comfort all who mourn,
and provide for those who grieve in Zion —
to bestow on them a crown of beauty
instead of ashes,
the oil of joy
instead of mourning,
and a garment of praise
instead of a spirit of despair.
They will be called oaks of righteousness,
a planting of the LORD
for the display of his splendour.

ISAIAH 61:1-3 NIV

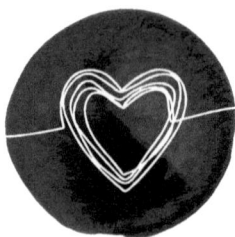

— *Father's Heart* —

When the troubles of this world come, and they will come, what will you choose to believe? My truth or the lies of the prince of heaviness?

My Spirit reflects My heart and nature.

I am good.

I am goodness.

There is none like Me. I have no beginning and no end.

When I tell you that I am good, it means there is nothing bad about Me.

Walking in My ways and choosing My truth instead of what you feel, see or experience in the natural world is a part of walking in the opposite spirit.

I love it when you spend time getting to know Me.

It is out of our relationship that you form a solid foundation for knowing whether something is from Me, or opposed to My heart.

Know Me, and you will know freedom.

The world would have you believe that this is not normal. They would have you think that you are broken for wanting something better. But I tell you that there is a way to walk in life that is higher and lovelier than you could ever have imagined!

It is time, My child, to recalibrate your design back to its original, pure and powerful structure.

Cast off those things that do not reflect My heart and My nature. They are not a good fit for you; they were never destined for you to carry or deal with alone. I tell you, walk in the opposite of what comes at you; give it a try.

If it is healthier and reflects My nature, what do you have to lose?

Burdens? Worry? Heaviness?

You were designed for so much more than what you are burdened by.

With Me, it is possible, My beloved, to have peace in times of angst.

With Me, it is possible to have love for someone even when they have crushed your heart.

With Me, it is possible to forgive the unforgivable and be free.

It is possible, it is possible, it IS possible!

All things are possible with Me.

I have a current available to you right now — a stream of living water.

OPPOSITE

Step into the cool, refreshing place of peace with Me.

*Dip your toe into the current that flows
with My life-giving Spirit.*

*Do not swim against My tide anymore, My child.
That way of swimming depletes your resources.*

*But I have a way for you to wade out into the depths
and swim, living in freedom, whatever comes at you.*

*Whatever the enemy throws at you is not
beyond you because I am with you.*

*I have plans that will shake off those things, lifting you
up to your rightful status—as an overcomer—with Me.*

*It's time to cast off those chains which have been hanging
around your neck—and dive into the waters which
bring life to your bones and sweetness to your song.*

*This is My current and My currency for You
because I love you and want you to be free.*

The sinful nature wants to do evil, which is just the opposite
of what the Spirit wants. And the Spirit gives us desires
that are the opposite of what the sinful nature desires.
These two forces are constantly fighting each other, so
you are not free to carry out your good intentions.

GALATIANS 5:17 NLT

You, dear children, are from God and have overcome them, because the one who is in you is greater than the one who is in the world.

1 JOHN 4:4 NIV

— *Prayer* —

Countercultural, loving Father,

Your ways are often opposite to how my natural self might feel.

Where others sow in hate, You encourage me to bring Your love.

Where the world pushes and pulls at me, You say, "Come, rest a while."

It all started with Your grace, loving me when I didn't deserve it, and You haven't stopped turning things on their head.

Where I have upset, You have joy,

Where I have questions and frustration, you have answers and strategies,

Where there is angst, You have oodles of peace available for me.

Whatever the problem, I believe You have a way through or out.

You crushed everything that might have come against me when Jesus died. He then rose from the dead, conquering death once and for all.

Nothing need scare, intimidate or crush me because You have redeemed it ALL.

Align my heart to Your truth that I might live in true freedom in You.

Amen.

XXXXX

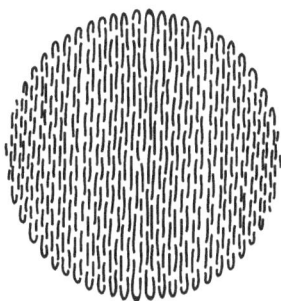

Chapter Four

BLESSING

See, I am setting before you today a blessing and a curse.

DEUTERONOMY 11:26 NASB 1995

The Lord bless you and keep you; the Lord make His face shine upon you and be gracious to you; the Lord lift up his countenance upon you and give you peace.

NUMBERS 6:24-26 ESV

Y ou are the ugliest, most awful strawberry I've ever seen. You are horrible, and I wish you weren't here. You are shrivelled, dry, and tasteless; and I hate you."

Oh, Lord, I hate talking like this.

This has to be one of the strangest things I'd ever been asked to do.

I placed the sandwich bag with the strawberry inside back down on the stone kitchen bench. The bag with its large "C" written on it glistened in the light.

Cursing.

Glancing at the second bag with a large letter "I" written in thick black marker on the front…

Ignore.

That strawberry laid quietly on the bench, untouched, unheard, unseen; it seemed disconnected from everything. Sitting unmoved, subtly sweating in its little bag, probably wondering why no one

"YOU ARE
THE UGLIEST,
MOST AWFUL
STRAWBERRY I'VE
EVER SEEN. YOU
ARE HORRIBLE,
AND I WISH
YOU WEREN'T
HERE. YOU ARE
SHRIVELLED, DRY,
AND TASTELESS;
AND I HATE YOU."

was eating it. Why was no one looking at it or enjoying it?

My eyes tracked to the third bag, the one I had been looking forward to interacting with. With a large letter "B" on the front, I took it in my hands and made my way around the corner (so the other strawberries didn't hear what I said to this one).

"You are the most beautiful strawberry in the world! I bless you. I bless you with plump, juiciness and bright colours. I love how you are made. You grew just the way you were meant to, and no other strawberry is as good as you. Bless you, precious strawberry, we love you."

It feels great to be speaking these kinds of things, rather than the other.

Its bright red skin seemed to glow with delight as I replaced it on the stone bench…and went about my day.

Yesterday was a strange one. A doctor's appointment and like the first bag, my speech was full of disappointment, complaint and lack. My week had been hard, and my doctor was a safe place to share all that was on my heart.

"The kids are arguing all the time and clashing.

I'm beyond tired and struggling physically. It's like everything is going really well with God and family and life. Then BOOM. Something happens and then my health stuff flares up.

The enemy always seems to get at me through my health."

Frustrated by the lack of breakthrough and forward movement, this became my focus. And with that focus came a flood of—"real" talk.

She sat in her chair, nodding occasionally, as she listened.

She waited patiently for me.

She didn't butt in or tell me I was wrong.

Instead, she took out a single square of note paper and began writing a list.

"After our time, I want you to head to the shops and pick up a punnet of strawberries. They need to be as fresh as possible, with at least three similar-looking strawberries inside."

"THE ENEMY ALWAYS SEEMS TO GET AT ME THROUGH MY HEALTH."

My head looked at her quizzically. "Why?"

"I have a family experiment I want you to do."

An internal groan swirled about inside my gut; *science has never been my thing.*

She'd written the instructions down for us, and as Craig and I headed home that afternoon, I found the questions come.

What is this about? What will happen? How does this relate to my healing? My betterment? Why has she asked us to do this?

She'd been so mysterious about the experiment and hadn't given anything away, which only served to make me question even further.

Her parting message, "There is power in your words, Karen."

I nodded in agreement and departed her office, thinking upon what she'd shared; intrigued to begin the experiment.

That night, as we collected three sandwich bags and our strawberries, none of us could have imagined what fruit this simple suggestion would bring.

Over the course of the week, we spoke words of blessing over one strawberry. We ignored another. And with the third, we spoke lack, negativity over it.

HER PARTING MESSAGE, "THERE IS POWER IN YOUR WORDS, KAREN."

One by one each family member headed into the pantry, picked up a bag and spoke to it in the next room. Then returned the bag to its original position. It was wonderful to see our family engaging with this experiment.

First-day observations: no change in any of the strawberries.

Second-day observations: we noted the cursed and ignored strawberries both looked a little soft. The blessed strawberry continued looking like it had just been picked from the patch.

Third-day observations: we noted the cursed strawberry had begun to lose some of its juice. *(Is that poor little thing crying?)*

The ignored strawberry looked very soft and squishy.

The blessed strawberry looked as good as if it had just been picked.

By the end of the fourth day, as I picked up the cursed strawberry bag, I noted it had cried all its juice, which pooled like a red puddle in the corner of the bag.

Squooshy, soft, and inedible.

I feel so sorry for it.

We did this! How horrible!

Glancing down at this squelched strawberry, I was reminded of the things I'd spoken against myself, especially during this time of affliction.

I cringed as I remembered speaking the same line, "The enemy always gets to me through my health."

The revelation of this little squashed strawberry was proving to be a convicting symbol of something so profound and deep.

Lord, I'm so sorry for saying that the enemy gets at me through my health. I agreed with this because it felt true, but it went against Your truth. Please forgive me. I renounce this curse I've spoken against myself; please lift it from me entirely in Jesus' name.

The ignored strawberry which had not been touched for the entire four days had also cried its juice, but this strawberry had also gone mouldy. The mold was all over the inside of the bag. This one reminded me of the children who are never held, never given loving words of encouragement. It reminded me of those lonely, bitter hearts who never have a kind word to say. They must feel like this strawberry.

My heart expanded with compassion and sorrow.

Poor thing; we did this too.

Picking up the blessed strawberry, I carefully opened the bag. Not knowing how it would feel, I hadn't even opened the other bags; they were too gross.

But this one…

No squooshed parts. No strawberry tears, no mold. After four days of positive talk and blessings, the berry was still good enough to eat: firm, plump, juicy, and delicious, looking as if it had just been picked.

It was perfect!

BLESSING

This is amazing!

The family were all greatly impacted by this experience, and I noted over the following days and weeks that we began to be more intentional about how we spoke to one another, what we said about ourselves, and others.

Thank You, God, for giving us a visual example of the power of blessing.

Bless those who persecute you; bless and do not curse.

ROMANS 12:14 NIV

I call heaven and earth to witness against you today, that I have set before you life and death, the blessing and the curse. So choose life in order that you may live, you and your descendants.

DEUTERONOMY 30:19 NASB

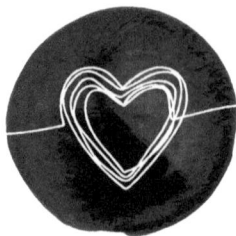

— Father's Heart —

My word is My blessing.

When you invite Me in, trusting Me with any situation, I will bring redemption to it.

It is My heart to bless.

I love to bless My children.

I love to show them the depths of My love for them.

Not only does My blessing make you feel a small portion of My love, but it helps deepen your trust.

When you choose to bless instead of curse, life is released.

I am life.

When you speak words of blessing over someone, I am released to work in them.

Blessing comes not as something deserved; it is a result of My grace.

I bless you—not because of what you do, but rather who you are in Me.

Trust Me to work all things for good.

When you choose to bless, the plans of any foe are obliterated, and they stand in confusion at the blessing.

Every curse that is upon you, I will turn for blessing.

Stand firm in My name. No matter what comes your way — know that I am always with you. You are blessed and will continue to be blessed.

Even during hard times, I am with you.

As I am with you — My abundance, love and answers are available to you.

These are all blessings.

When you feel like complaining, gossiping, speaking words of discontent...Stop.

Talk to Me about your worries. Invite Me into your circumstance and concern. Become aware of the atmosphere around and in you. As you become more aware of Me, you have an opportunity to see My life-giving perspective of what you are going through.

Every word you might have spoken in lack, now choose to declare in love.

Declare blessing in My name, and I will show you just how powerful I am.

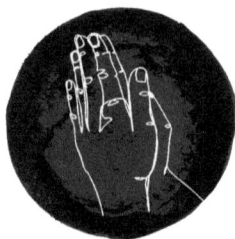

— Prayer —

Thank You, Lord, for being One who LOVES to bless.

I am so grateful that You bless all aspects of my life.

Bless this life You've given me.

Bless my home, work and play.

Bless our relationship, Lord God.

Bless my hopes, my dreams and future.

Thank You for resourcing me for Your good plans.

Lord, please show me the way forward, that I may be in step with Your blessing, plans and calling.

Lord, I ask You to encourage me with confirming signs along the way.

Help me to keep watch for opportunities to step into blessing. Let my words, thoughts and actions reflect Your heartbeat of blessing.

Father, bless me and those You place in my sphere of influence.

Help me to know my worth and the depth of Your love for me.

Thank You for the good gifts You give us each day.

Amen.

XXXXX

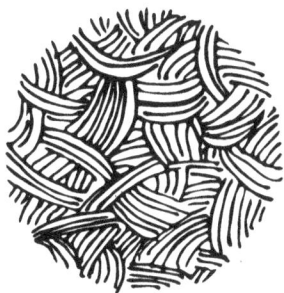

Chapter Five

PROPHETIC WORDS

But the one who prophesies speaks to people for
their strengthening, encouraging and comfort.

1 CORINTHIANS 14:3 NIV

Now I wish that you all spoke in tongues, but even more that you would prophesy; and greater is one who prophesies than one who speaks in tongues, unless he interprets, so that the church may receive edifying.

1 CORINTHIANS 14:5 NASB 1995

Waiting online for David Wagner to join the zoom meeting, my body buzzed.

It has been a hard slog, Lord. Leaping back into study has been huge. Is my body going to hold up?

Summer had been intensely hot, which meant I was dehydrated most of the time, physical flow on effects ensued.

It was February, but the whole summer had been challenging.

Christmas had been a dud.

We hadn't gone to church for the first time in years because everyone was so cranky and exhausted from the end-of-year strain.

On top of everything else, my doctor was exploring whether I had glandular fever.

CHRISTMAS HAD
BEEN A DUD.

Stairway School of Transformation and completing my Certificate 4 in Ministry and Theology was proving exciting and exhausting.

Thankfully, I can study online, but what will today be like?

We'd begun the year studying the prophetic; new language for me. The first few weeks of study had covered the biblical basis for prophecy, and today, we were receiving a prophetic word. I had been learning that the prophetic was not mystical or magical, but at its core — the giving and receiving of encouragements from God.

Encouragement — I am IN!

Waiting for the meeting to begin, the nerves began to ping around in my system.

Lord, what if You say something through this guy about my health?

What if You don't? What if I hear something I'm not ready to hear?

Be still, My child, you won't be disappointed.

I am weary, Lord, and don't know what to expect. Please protect my heart. I've had so many harsh words spoken; it's been such a hard time since before Christmas. So much has been stolen.

I've got you, and I've got this; there is no need to fear.

Immediately, as I heard this, the screen flickered, and David appeared, introducing himself to my friend and me.

He then began praying a tender prayer, asking for Holy Spirit to bring His life words to us both.

David began sharing what God had placed on his heart for my friend.

That's incredible and so timely for her.

I wouldn't have believed it unless I had heard it with my own ears. He had nailed her heart completely.

Instead of reassuring me, his words only served to increase my nervousness.

A sense of preparing for disappointment tried to infiltrate my fatigued brain.

David began prophesying and sharing all that God gave Him for me.

"Karen, I saw the Lord putting things in your arms; the things were precious like babies and things that were somewhat vulnerable."

Wow!!! Oh, Lord…I've always had strangers share their lives and problems with me. Often people who were fragile.

It's so rare that I don't meet those who are walking through tough. This is amazing!

He often gave me life words and encouragement that seemed to speak to them. (Unbeknownst to me, this was being prophetic!)

"KAREN, I SAW THE LORD PUTTING THINGS IN YOUR ARMS; THE THINGS WERE PRECIOUS LIKE BABIES AND THINGS THAT WERE SOMEWHAT VULNERABLE."

David, who had not met me before today, who didn't know a thing about me apart from what God had showed him, continued, speaking reassuring words about my healing.

Wow! I'd come here with so much mystery and many questions.

The words washed over me, addressing every question I had brought to God before the meeting had begun.

You are amazing, Lord! Thank You!

As I sat there with my mouth open in utter surprise and delight, I endeavoured to drink it all in. Finally, David shared a word which spoke to something only God can have known.

PROPHETIC WORDS

He stopped for a moment, and said, "I am hearing a Christmas song playing…when heaven and nature sing."

He continued, "I feel like it's going to feel like Christmas all year to you."

My heart began to dance and sing, as I envisioned what it might feel like to have Christmas all year round.

Even speaking to my disappointment about our most recent Christmas season.

God was restoring it in full to me.

My mind danced with joy.

> GOD WAS RESTORING IT IN FULL TO ME.

My body buzzed with delight.

My heart sang with intense celebration at all that had been shared.

This was to be the first of many words God gave me during this season.

Connecting with like-hearted prophetic people — the God poetry of bringing timely words of encouragement, strategy, comfort, whatever He knew someone needed.

Through this special morning God had opened the prophetic chapter for me and gave me language for something I had been doing for decades.

I finally felt like I'd discovered what I'd been made for, and I knew I was never going back to life without this precious key.

We also have the prophetic message as something completely reliable, and you will do well to pay attention to it, as to a light shining in a dark place, until the day dawns and the morning star rises in your hearts. Above all, you must understand that no prophecy of Scripture came about by the prophet's own interpretation of things. For prophecy never had its origin in the human will, but prophets, though human, spoke from God as they were carried along by the Holy Spirit.

2 PETER 1:19-21 NIV

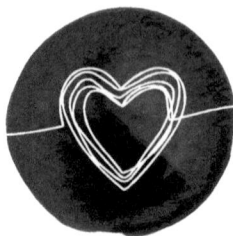

— Father's Heart —

My words never return to Me empty.

Are you weary, dry, or wandering in the wilderness of life?

*Do you wonder where I am and what I would say
about all that you are walking through?*

*I have sweet words of hope for you—words that will be like
honey to your soul and a healing balm for your heart.*

*My words always reflect My heart of love for you and
My desire to bring you good things that invest life.*

You need never fear. The words I say are always for your good.

*I have plans for a hope and future for you, and
My words will always reflect this intention.*

*Prophetic words are simply words of encouragement
and instruction for you. They are markers,
helpers bringing life-giving strategies.*

They are not orders or commands; that isn't My heart or nature.

*My words are invitations to partner with My heart. Will you join
with My plan for your life? Will you say yes to the things I have for
you? Will you choose the things that I know will bring the best?*

I desire this for you, My precious one, because I love you.

Sometimes these words will come through My Word. They might be brought through My children. Other times they might be given creatively.

The way of communication is not as important as the message I am releasing to you.

Keep watch. Be aware of Me in the everyday. Ask questions.

Look out for Me, beloved. I am not hidden as you sometimes believe.

I am bringing you messages of hope and delight constantly.

It's My message melody to draw you closer to Myself and invest the very things that you need to take the next step. I am with you.

Stop for a moment and become aware of Me in the noise. Be still before me and pick up My peace. From this awareness, you will begin to see Me in all things.

Life will unfold before you in miraculous and empowering ways.

My words draw you nearer to Me—anything else isn't Me.

Look for the things that enable us to connect authentically with one another. As you become aware of Me, you will learn to recognize My sound, My nature, and My heart.

I get great delight as we connect with one another in this way, My precious child.

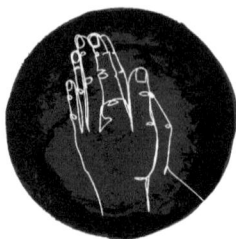

— *Prayer* —

Father, Jesus, and Holy Spirit,

Thank You for speaking to me, for always having something good to say.

Thank You for bringing messages of hope through this area of prophetic words.

Your encouragement is always welcome in my life.

Please entwine our hearts, making it so that I'd always desire to connect with You and listen to Your instruction.

Thank You that prophecy is—at its base—listening to You and sharing what You say. Thank You that this is available to all.

Help me discern what is from You, embracing these words and releasing anything else.

I'm so relieved that You are not limited by my limitations—but use my willing heart to speak life to others. Bless those who have brought Your timely words through words of prophecy to me, in Jesus' name.

Amen.

XXXXX

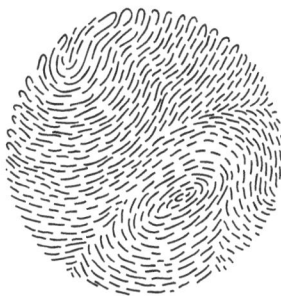

Chapter Six

PROPHETIC ACTS

Having said these things, he spit on the ground and made mud with the saliva. Then he anointed the man's eyes with the mud and said to him, "Go, wash in the pool of Siloam" (which means Sent). So he went and washed and came back seeing.

JOHN 9:6-7 ESV

And so it was, when Moses held up his hand, that Israel prevailed; and when he let down his hand, Amalek prevailed. But Moses' hands *became* heavy; so they took a stone and put *it* under him, and he sat on it. And Aaron and Hur supported his hands, one on one side, and the other on the other side; and his hands were steady until the going down of the sun.

EXODUS 17:11- 12

S tanding at the gate of our land, everything looked bare.

Are we meant to even build here, Lord?

We'd been battling through for years, endeavouring to get something built, but we kept hitting brick walls.

A car pulled up, and a lady hopped out. I recognized our neighbour from down the road. She'd come to tend to her miniature horses, which were agisted on our property.

"How are you going with the planning process?" she asked.

"It's been really tough actually, darlin. They are making it difficult to build here, but I'm sure it'll work out,"
I responded.

"I've always thought this land was cursed."

I was floored.

This woman, who didn't have a faith, felt our land, where our home would be built — was cursed.

"I'VE ALWAYS
THOUGHT THIS
LAND WAS
CURSED."

Clenching my teeth, trying to stop myself from reacting, I asked, "What makes you think that?"

She responded, "There have been two owners of this land that I know of, and no one has been able to build on it. The last owners ended up having to sell because of health issues."

As she said this, my skin crawled.

I hate the idea of anything being cursed, but especially the site of our future home.

My spirit became righteously angry about it.

The following day I was driving to a meeting and found myself with half an hour of "free" time.

> **I LOOKED AT THE TWO AND A HALF ACRES OF LAND BEFORE ME, AND I COULDN'T SEE A SINGLE BIRD.**

As I headed toward my appointment, I began dreaming what I might do with this extra time.

Without thinking I found myself turning the car toward the block of land.

It's on the way, I've got time.

As I drove toward the block, I sensed these words in my heart.

Give Me the land, My child. Consecrate the land to Me and watch what happens.

I don't know what this means, but whatever You want me to do, I am in!

Yesterday's conversation was still playing on my mind.

Maybe God wants to address it?

I pulled up the drive a little, jumped the fence, and walked to the top of the hill. As I strolled, I noted all the birds on the neighbour's land. I love birds and notice them everywhere I go. God had often used their ways to speak to me.

This got me thinking.

I looked at the two and a half acres of land before me, and I couldn't see a single bird.

We had some wonderfully large gum trees and scrub around the boundaries of the land, but not one bird could be seen.

Where are the birds?

Where are our birds? Have I ever seen birds here?

No, I don't think I so.

Lord, what's going on with that?

He reminded me of what I'd come there to do.

Worship Me. Give Me the land, and thank Me for it. Do whatever I bring to your mind to do.

I continued to pace the hill with water bottle in hand. I organically began to sing.

Singing over the land and giving it back to the Lord.

"This is Your land, Lord. Every speck of dirt, every blade of grass, every molecule of dirt, every drop of water, every air particle is Yours and Yours alone." I sang out at the top of my lungs.

I declared life over the land.

Any Scripture that came to mind, I declared out loud to the atmosphere.

I blessed every part and gave God my thanks for this precious moment with Him. I'd never done anything like this before, but worshiping this way, in His way—felt great.

I sang and danced before Him.

I probably look like a fool, but I don't care.

He then showed me a picture of me opening the lid of my bottle and pouring the water upon the land.

So I did exactly as He had shown me.

As I did this, it felt as if I was consecrating the land to Him. Whatever happened, it was His to do with as He pleased.

The moment the water bottle emptied, sunlight flashed brilliantly across my eyes.

My sight was drawn heavenward, as I saw three majestic broadwinged white birds. As I looked at them flying in unison, their wings expanded even farther, gliding the currents.

My heart flew with them.

I PROBABLY LOOK
LIKE A FOOL, BUT
I DON'T CARE.

I felt a joy return to the space that had once been so heavy within me. And all that the lady had shared felt redeemed.

Watching these birds fly high above our property was pure sunshine for my soul. Clouds above, absolute peace and birds releasing their call above. They were the first birds I had seen since we had bought the block. Amazing!

My skin tingled with delight—our first birds!

A holy moment of pure joy and freedom.

I knew something significant had happened.

He'd given me an instruction, a small whisper of an idea, and I'd part-nered with it. I'd not felt this invested freedom in my spirit before.

(This single act of obedience, a moment in time, broke something over the land, and since this time, birds flock to our home: ducks, black and white cockatoos, rosellas, magpies, ibises, eagles, hawks, parrots and many more.)

This simple act seemed to align the land with His heart. The antici-pation I now felt because of this small act of faith drew me to want more of this kind of encounter with Him and His freeing power of blessing.

And as we stayed many days, a certain prophet named Agabus came down from Judea. When he had come to us, he took Paul's belt, bound his own hands and feet, and said, "Thus says the Holy Spirit, 'So shall the Jews at Jerusalem bind the man who owns this belt, and deliver him into the hands of the Gentiles.' "

ACTS 21:10-12 NKJV

PROPHETIC ACTS

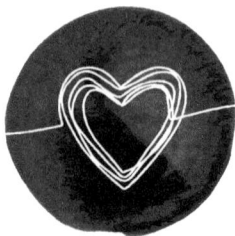

— Father's Heart —

Trust Me, for I am trustworthy.

I have so much for us to do together. Some things will involve you acting in ways that are not comfortable or make logical sense.

I am bigger than human logic. I am greater than what is seen with the human eye.

My heart is for you, not against you, My child.

I will not ask you to do anything beyond your capability or what I have resourced you for.

When I ask you to do something in faith, trust Me to partner with you as you step forward in obedience.

If I have said it, if I have promised it, I will do this for you. Trust Me to know what you need.

Sometimes I will ask you to intercede on behalf of a situation or person in your life.

I will highlight them to you. No matter how silly it may seem, trust Me and be obedient to what I have placed on your heart to do.

*Then release it to Me fully and move
on with the rest of the day.*

*Celebrate and thank Me for what I am doing because
I am always doing something. That is the truth.*

*Many of you fear the people you see and
what they might think of you.*

Do not try to seek human approval, but Mine.

The truth is you already have My approval.

I know how amazing you are!

*Nothing you do can make Me love you
any more than I do right now.*

*I love you completely—100 percent—and
have done since the beginning of time.*

*By choosing to be obedient to My call, our relationship
is placed first and foremost in your life.*

It brings Me joy to see you flourishing in union with Me.

*In faith, prophetic acts welcome more of Me
into a situation and a greater revelation
of Myself into a person, place or thing.*

*I look forward to releasing My truth into a
situation, displaying My glory and perfection
within it, creating poetry before your eyes,
astounding the eyes and hearts of the scoffers.*

*The truth of My heavenly realm infiltrates
the natural world through acts of faith.*

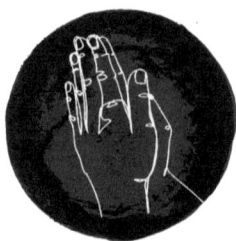

— Prayer —

Father, Your ways are majestic and wonderful to me.

Thank You for Your creativity and Your Holy Spirit who loves to be part of prophetic acts.

I do not always understand the intricacies of these, but I do know that You work in powerful ways through them.

You have blessed, healed, given freedom and spoken through them.

Lord, some of these things seemed bizarre when the idea came, but anything which aligns with Your Word and loving nature is never to be feared.

Father, I am in awe of You and each act that You invite me to participate in.

Soften my heart to these things of You, Father.

Thank You for continuing to teach me about Yourself through this key.

Thank You for loving, faith-filled acts that invite Your life-changing power into a situation.

I love Your ways.

Amen.

XXXXX

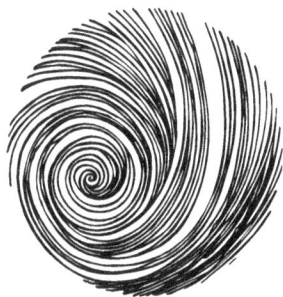

Chapter Seven

JOY

Until now you have not asked for anything in my name.
Ask and you will receive, and your joy will be complete.

JOHN 16:24 NIV

Then he said to them, "Go your way. Eat the fat and drink sweet wine and send portions to anyone who has nothing ready, for this day is holy to our Lord. And do not be grieved, for the joy of the Lord is your strength."

NEHEMIAH 8:10 ESV

S truggle city had been the tone of the week; symptoms galore and life stress had both escalated.

How long will it be, Lord? When will this end?

The pain was excruciating at times.

Over the past few months, I'd had several people pray for me. And the theme of each was joy…the very thing I felt nothing of.

I don't feel joyful. I can't even feign happiness.

How am I supposed to be joyful when I am in pain?

Each prayer seemed to prick the issue that was at hand, leaving me frustrated and full of angst.

How do I get joy? That was the question I struggled with in my depths.

How can I be joyful in pain?

HOW AM I SUPPOSED TO BE JOYFUL WHEN I AM IN PAIN?

How can I be joyful while watching other people do the things I should be doing as a mum?

How can I be joyful when the finances are dropping?

How can I be joyful when there seem to be no answers—only questions?

Joy was regularly spoken about in God's Word.

He kept bringing verses that spoke about joy, placing them in front of me.

Have Joy.

Joy is your strength.

Consider it pure joy.

Joy comes in the morning.

It seemed joy was inescapable for me in this season.

I had gone up to the front at church for prayer regarding my health so many times I had lost count. Each time I went up, I received the joy-themed messages. As people prayed, they spoke the very things God had been saying to me in my journaling: "Be still," and "Have joy."

So frustrating. They keep saying have joy—like it's a choice! What am I supposed to do with this, Lord?

As precious-hearted prayers shared these joy encouragements with me, it felt like rubbing salt into the wound.

Until finally, over the past few weeks, on at least eight different occasions, the same words were spoken: "I see you full of joy!"

I don't know what they were seeing, but it felt as far from me as the moon and the stars.

I'm DONE! What does this mean, Lord? Why are these people saying the same thing? Am I missing something?

If it's You, then bring me joy. If they are getting it wrong, please protect my heart from these words. If it's me, help me to see the next step. I need to understand what they are saying.

Obviously, something was in the message I wasn't comprehending, and my frustration continued to grow, as did my questions.

How am I supposed to be joyful when I am so physically unwell? Will joy ever be a part of my life again? Can the two co-exist?

Answers came when we received an invitation to a 48-hour prayer event.

I FOUGHT THE URGE TO LAUGH OUT LOUD.

The gathering sounded wonderful to me. Desperate for difference, Craig, the family and I went. We spent a couple of hours talking to God in different ways. We selected rolled-up Bible verses from a large well. Unsurprisingly, mine were about joy. We received verses in other ways, and every single time throughout the night, mine was about joy.

There was an opportunity to go forward as a family to receive a prophetic word. Unsurprisingly, once again, the words for me were ALL about joy.

"I sense that God is saying you have such a joyful spirit."

Something broke inside and instead of being frustrated or angry, I fought the urge to laugh out loud.

This is getting so ridiculous.

Each verse I received that day related to joy, the prophetic word was about joy and as we headed toward home, I felt an emptiness.

How can I be joyful when I'm unable to "do" anything?

That night, God gave me a dream that helped to answer the internal conflict.

I dreamt about the apostle Paul.

I saw some of his experiences one after the other—storms, shipwrecks, chains, and prisons. The dream was intense and wonderful. As I awakened, one question rattled around in my heart:

How could Paul go through all those things and still be able to sing about the goodness of God and revel in joy?

It seemed impossible for a human to be like that.

Lord, I don't know how it happened, but I want that too!

JOY DOESN'T COME FROM YOU; IT'S NOT SOMETHING YOU CREATE.

As I journaled out all that was on my heart, finally broaching the inner frustrations about joy, He revealed some truth that opened it up.

Joy doesn't come from you; it's not something you create.

It comes as a by-product of an awareness of Me.

By being with Me, you will experience joy. You will carry joy. You will have joy!

Joy isn't happiness because happiness comes and goes like the wind, but My joy remains. You have believed that joy is the same as being happy, My beloved. Joy doesn't leave, because I am always with you, and I am Your source of joy.

As I read what He'd written, the penny dropped, and I realised that those prayers, those words, they were all revealing the very thing God wanted to restore to me.

Over the following weeks and months, I noticed that I indeed DID have joy. It had not disappeared. Joy was not absent or paralysed as I'd once felt. My awareness of it had been awakened. Joy was alive and well. And this was cause for celebration.

Thank You, Lord!

You have enlarged the nation and increased their joy;
they rejoice before you as people rejoice at the harvest,
as warriors rejoice when dividing the plunder.

ISAIAH 9:3 CEB

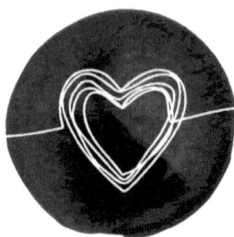

— Father's Heart —

Joy is My song to you, beloved.

It is a way that I love you with the language of heaven.

Joy is what I use to pour My everything upon you.

*It is a door to break through and learn
the rhythms of My heartbeat.*

*Joy is powerful because it is Me. I want My
children to see and experience Me fully.*

*It is My way for you to encounter complete
freedom, release, and life!*

*When circumstances come and endeavour
to take you off the right path, My joy can
release everything you need to combat it.*

Joy is My gift to you, and it is available to you as a constant.

As you step into My rest, you WILL encounter Me.

*My heartbeat never fails to release joy,
especially in this place of communion.*

*As you step into and are reassured of
who you are, joy is present.*

As you know Me more, joy is expanded.

As you learn to trust Me in whatever comes, joy is available.

Joy is a power tool for life. It allows you to walk through the tough and remain centred in Me.

Joy breeds My hope. It's the anchor which holds you steadfast in faith — and in life.

The world will tell you, "Strive for happiness." I say to you, "Strive for more of Me." Then you will have all you need and more.

As the embers of joy are stoked, it doesn't take much for those tiny sparks to become a wildfire of courage, confidence, peace and inner delight.

Flames which help to combat the barbs of the enemy, fear, anxiety, worry and whatever comes to throw you off your track.

My joy supersedes all fear.

Invite Me into every moment and ask for joy.

Then keep watch as it will not be far away.

Desire My joy! Reach out for it, look for it, and learn to recognise it.

It is easier to find joy in the "be still" with Me, but it is always available.

Turn your eyes to Me afresh, My beloved. The choice to look up will invest faith, which builds trust as you encounter Me.

Know that the more you know Me, the greater you will walk in joy.

JOY

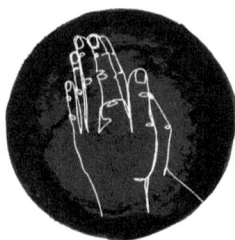

— *Prayer* —

Joyful Father,

I can't tell You how much I love to be joyful; it's such a delight to be in that sweet space with You, Father.

I know You long for me to live in Your provision of joy.

I don't always feel joyful in all circumstances, but with Your help, my eyes and heart can attune to it.

Help me to ask for what I need and then receive what You give in return.

Thank You for the apostle Paul and the way his life reflects that joy is possible in my life, whatever I walk through.

Thank You for Your precious Son, Jesus. His life shines so brightly to me that joy is possible even with the heaviness of humankind on His shoulders. It is achievable and possible in You.

Thank You that joy is never absent from me because where You are I have access to it.

Increase my awareness of joy in life, sweet Jesus.

Amen.

XXXXX

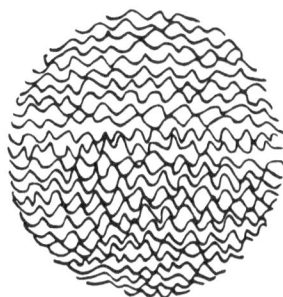

Chapter Eight

INTERCESSION

I urge, then, first of all, that petitions, prayers, intercession
and thanksgiving be made for all people — for kings
and all those in authority, that we may live peaceful
and quiet lives in all godliness and holiness.

1 TIMOTHY 2:1-2 NIV

He was amazed to see that no one intervened to help the oppressed. So he himself stepped in to save them with his strong arm, and his justice sustained him.

ISAIAH 59:16 NLT

'm sick of myself and my problems. Every day runs into the next.

As I pulled dirty dishes from our burgundy bench top and swished them around the hot water, I felt myself washing each dish with an energy that reflected my inner frustration.

Desperate to see something shift—something change.

Is this IT, Lord?

Each day feels the same-except I'm not the same.

I'm trying to work out who I am now. I can't do what I once could. I'm trying to work out what I'm supposed to be doing.

The phone vibrated on the upper bench and then moved across it toward me. I grabbed it with my pink gloved hand, flicking water from it.

A BABY LAY
IN HOSPITAL
STRUGGLING
TO SURVIVE.

It was my sister sharing a call for prayer.

A baby lay in hospital struggling to survive.

This message was an urgent cry for help.

My mumma heart swelled with intensity as I read it.

This is full on.

Instead of bursting into tears at the thought of what the family was going through, my body responded very differently to what was my "normal."

The second I saw the message, I felt a wave of energy course through my veins as I felt a loud, "NO" cry from my spirit.

"This is NOT happening."

An uncharacteristic boldness was instilled deep in my heart.

Time to take this to God.

My heart beat fast as the energy burst out. I found myself pacing around our kitchen island bench.

"Oh, Father, we need You! Protect and heal this little one. Tend to every part that is not aligned with Your design. Heal him, Lord.

Bring down his temperature to normal levels.

Restore the energy that is rightfully his.

Touch every organ with Your healing touch, in Jesus' name."

I found that the more I prayed, the more enthusiastically my arms pointed and moved, as if to express all that He had placed on my heart.

"We declare life into his fragile body. In fact, strengthen him. Lift fragility from him, Jesus. We speak life into him. Life. Life. Life."

Time passed quickly…who knows how long.

I am tired of illness.

I am weary of death.

An internal courage was present, to "go into bat" for this little stranger. Every thought, no matter how small, I spoke out, prayed for, declared, and asked God for it all. He prompted me to pray for the parents—the doctors and medical staff, and even the hospital atmosphere.

As I declared life to his body systems, I sensed things moving. So real, as if I was seeing it unfold before my eyes. Things physically shifting in the hospital room, the staff, the machines, the cells of his body. It was all coming into alignment.

Peace.

My pacing ceased.

The righteous anger eased.

IT FELT...DONE.

Internal peace reigned within.

It felt...done.

As if God had put His seal upon the prayer, and I could let it go.

And once I'd prayed all I sensed—peace came, and the intensity subsided.

This little man is going to live.

The passion I felt for that little one was outside of myself. I didn't know the child, their family, or the church they belonged to. I didn't know the parents. I didn't even know the full details, but God did.

He was calling His saints to intercede for this baby. As I did, God brought peace to my spirit and settled the righteous anger and energy that surged through me only moments before.

INTERCESSION

I received a follow-up message soon after: the little boy was going to be okay. In fact, miraculously, he had turned a corner and was now recovering! Praise God!

In this experience, I felt God offer something fresh to me that was to be a fun and exciting part of my future. I enjoyed the experience of praying on behalf of another. Allowing God to show me who, what and where to pray and then following His lead.

It felt good to be able to give once again despite my limitations. This was finally something I could do!

Again I say to you, if two of you agree on earth about anything they ask, it will be done for them by my Father in heaven. For where two or three are gathered in my name, there am I among them.

MATTHEW 18:19-20 ESV

Seek the welfare of the city where I have sent
you into exile and pray to the Lord on its behalf;
for in its welfare you will have welfare.

JEREMIAH 29:7 NASB 1995

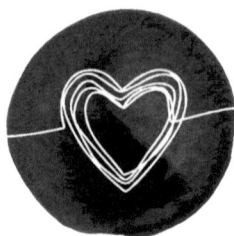

— Father's Heart —

*Cry out to Me on behalf of others. Sing
to Me of the things that burden.*

*Speak to Me, telling of the things that bring heaviness to
your heart, and I will meet you and lighten the load.*

*I will empower you to intercede on behalf of
others; all that you sense from Me.*

Trust Me with the things that are too big for words.

Let Me make a heavenly exchange as you hand them over.

*Bring Me the things which trouble your thoughts, emotions and
heart — start telling Me about them — in whatever way you wish.*

*Write, speak, dance, sing, draw, or allow My
Spirit to speak on your behalf in tongues.*

*As you release these things to Me, the realisation of Who
I am will be revealed to you to a greater measure.*

*As you acknowledge Who I am in it, then My great power
is released, both in the situation and within you.*

*You will see My Spirit transform the very things I have placed
upon your heart. I allowed these things so you would come
and share them with Me, enabling you and those around you*

*to stand in awe of My presence, My power and My ability
to do immeasurably more than you perceive or hope for.*

Have faith; I am always working.

*Intercession allows My heartbeat to be displayed and felt—by
the one—the one who matters more than anything else to Me.*

I allow this so you can see more of Me in the world.

I want you to know and experience Me in all things.

I want you to understand how much you matter to Me.

I want you to catch the heartbeat I have for others.

*I want you to receive a greater understanding and experience of
Who I am and the impact I can have in the world through you.*

*I have allowed certain burdens to impact your
heart to build intimacy between us and increase
compassion for others. Compassion is a key to unlock
so much. Encounters like this build your faith.*

*When you step out and intercede for another, the
love I have for you surges through you into the
spiritual atmosphere of this world and beyond.*

My Spirit loves to flow through these times of togetherness.

*When you intercede on behalf of another, it is a
step of faith, and I will not disappoint.*

*I love it when you come, walk, and trust Me with
something that might have initially troubled you.*

*I love to exchange the things of this world for
the heavenly things of My kingdom.*

*Trust Me, beloved. Come to Me heavy and fully
laden, and I will give you rest (Matthew 11:28). My
Word and leading will never return to Me void.*

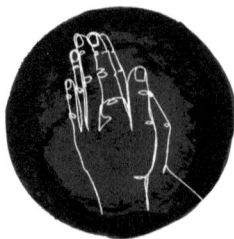

— Prayer —

*O Father, what a privilege to come during this
time of hardship and intercede for others.*

*Thank You for what You have shown me of Yourself. You
LOVE it when I pray, especially as Your Spirit leads.*

*Surely this is the greatest privilege: to pray and
impact another through Your loving will.*

Father, I want to be part of Your story more often.

*I want to pray the very heartbeat of You and feel the
desires of Your heart. Make them mine also, Father.*

Help me to notice and then embrace the things of Your heart.

*Thank You for being such a loving,
faithful God of breakthrough.*

*You have shown me this key of intercession and the power
it has to bring life and healing. And as I pray for others
miraculously my own situation is often touched.*

*Show me how and what to pray, reveal what Jesus is
interceding, and then release me to pray in the same way.*

In Jesus' name, amen.

XXXXX

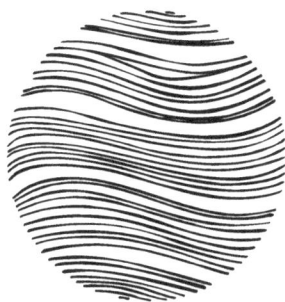

Chapter Nine

LOOKING BEYOND MYSELF

The generous will prosper; those who refresh
others will themselves be refreshed.

PROVERBS 11:25 NLT

So encourage each other and build each other up, just as you are already doing.

1 THESSALONIANS 5:11 NLT

He'd arrived at 8am sharp.

A cool wintry Melbourne morning. Being so early, the brain fog was like an old Holden Ute: the key clicks, the engine gasps, trying to turn over and finally spark to life — struggling to awaken.

Bed hair. Body weary. I sat at the kitchen table, eating some poached eggs and pears, trying to replenish after a task-heavy week, desperately needing some good, uninterrupted sleep and people-free days.

Today, however, this was not an option. Here he was, John, the firebox man, with thick, brown, slightly wavy hair, in his late twenties, lanky, with kind eyes and a warm smile. Friendly, and as it turns out, an absolute master in the installation of woodfire boxes.

Complaints tattered off like machine gun rapid fire within my mind.

I don't feel like having people in my home, Lord. I wish this wasn't happening today. I want to switch off for a bit from noise and people. The calendar has been so full, I just need a day's reprieve. Please let him go about his day and let me do mine.

John, with his tile-cutting tools, drills and hammers, worked away in the background. The sound reverberated throughout the house.

He's in my space—the space where my head needs peace and quiet.

John went about his work over the course of the morning, laying the hearth, positioning the soon-to-be sweet little wood box for lazy, toasty Sunday afternoons.

Aaahhh, won't that be lovely.

As I dreamt of "no rush," no scurry, agend-free time being warmed by the fire. Before I knew it, midday had arrived…lunchtime.

John gingerly knocked on the door and entered the house. "Could I borrow some water, please?" as he held up his two-minute noodle cup with a friendly grin.

Mood improved, I laughingly responded, "I can do better than that. You can have some!"

AS THE KETTLE BOILED, HE SAT ON THE KITCHEN STOOL BEHIND THE BENCH, AND WE STARTED CHATTING LIKE OLD FRIENDS.

As the kettle boiled, he sat on the kitchen stool behind the bench, and we started chatting like old friends.

No topics were off the agenda for John; he was proving to be a curious and thoughtful fella. The clock hands moved quickly past the hour.

Before I knew it, the subject of God came up.

The kettle bubbled and boiled and eventually clicked, alerting me it had finished its job. Pouring the water into the noodle cup, the conversation continued to roll with ease.

A wide grin spread across his lips. "You sound like my wife," he casually commented.

"How is that?" I enquired.

"Oh, you know, she goes to church sometimes. She's religious, like you."

Without skipping a beat, I responded, "I don't really consider myself religious, actually."

He looked at me, questioning what this response meant.

"I consider myself more *spiritual*. Religious, to me, means a whole lot of rules and regulations but, for me, spiritual is relational. My relationship with God is just that—a friendship. I talk to Him about the things going on in my life, and then I listen to what He might want to say to me. He talks to us all in our own ways. Ways we understand."

He nodded. "I think my wife is like that," adding, "I don't think I'm that spiritual either. I'm just not made that way, I suppose." His eyes dropped to the floor, downcast as the words left his lips.

My spirit grieved at his last comment; like a thorn, it panged in my heart.

Oh Lord, Lord. This is so wrong. He is spiritual. Please don't let him leave without meeting You.

"What kind of things make your wife spiritual?" I asked, offering a fork to John now that his noodles were brewing.

He took the fork from my hand and stirred the noodles as they softened inside the cup. "My wife kneels by her bed each night and prays with her hands together. I just leave her be when she's like that."

Maybe he's not meant to be like his wife.

That's right! He's not meant to be like her.

The penny dropped.

He thinks being spiritual is about kneeling to pray, leadlight windows and men in funny outfits chanting in large cathedrals.

My spirit leapt about as this light-bulb epiphany zipped in. "John, maybe you're not meant to be like your wife."

HE THINKS BEING SPIRITUAL IS ABOUT KNEELING TO PRAY, LEADLIGHT WINDOWS AND MEN IN FUNNY OUTFITS CHANTING IN LARGE CATHEDRALS.

He laughed and said, "You got that right! What do you mean, though?"

A picture of John popped into my mind's eye. He was in the middle of the bush, surrounded by scrub and large gum trees. They overhung the smoky fire which had been burning all night. John sat in the early hours of the morning in his camp chair. Hot drink in mug, warming his hands as he sat watching the flicker of flames. He was alone, as the thick morning mist and brisk air hung about. Motorbikes sat in the background, and half a dozen tents encircled the campfire.

I watched in the picture, as John looked around at the surroundings, appreciating nature and its beauty. Listening. Looking. Taking in the peace and enjoying the quiet. Holy ground for John.

This is John's cathedral! Oh Lord, Lord, thank You! This is amazing!

I shared the picture with him. "What if God speaks to you while you're in the bush, enjoying some motorbiking with mates? Sitting by the fire, appreciating the beautiful surroundings. What if this is how He connects with you, John?"

His eyes grew wide with delight. "That's my kind of church!" he cheered.

All went silent for a moment or two as he processed this idea, turning it over in his mind. I could almost see the cogs turning, as he stirred the now-soft noodles, almost ready to eat.

His eyes widened with amazement as the picture I'd described rang true. "How did you know that? I do like camping and motorbiking."

Oh, Lord, You are AMAZING. Thank You!

"I do sit by the campfire in the bush and look at what's around me. I love it. I go all the time and it's just like that. That's amazing. How did you know that?"

My eyes teared up a little as I saw John being wowed.

"That's God, John. He is the only One Who could have known that. You know that I can't have known that. I don't think you coming here today was a mistake. He wanted you to know how much He wants to talk with you." I quickly added, "And to tell you it's okay that you're not like your wife."

We both laughed.

"I like that. I reckon you might be right," he responded thoughtfully.

John went outside not long after, having consumed the noodles and been encouraged by God through a personal picture of his life. He laid the hearth, cut the holes in the roof and ceiling, and positioned the flue. He moved the firebox into position and sealed it all up.

HIS EYES GREW WIDE WITH DELIGHT. "THAT'S MY KIND OF CHURCH!" HE CHEERED.

Throughout the afternoon, he would occasionally poke his head in and ask another question or make another comment. Never had a tradesman done such an honourable job in our home.

What a gift the day had been!

No, it wasn't what I'd felt like today. I had wanted to remain in my own little world, but God had other ideas. I could have shut him out. I could have said no, but what an adventure I'd have missed out on if I had!

By the end of the day John had cleaned up every speck of mess, collected his tools, waved goodbye, and headed home to "tell his wife all about it."

Hubby Craig and I snuggled in front of our new little firebox. It was cosy warm. I shared what God had done with the day — a day where I'd chosen to say yes, and the problems of my world shrank because of God growing in John's.

Remember this: the person who sows sparingly
will also reap sparingly and the person who sows
generously will also reap generously.

2 CORINTHIANS 9:6 HCSB

Love must be sincere. Hate what is evil; cling to what is good. Be devoted to one another in love. Honor one another above yourselves. Never be lacking in zeal, but keep your spiritual fervor, serving the Lord. Be joyful in hope, patient in affliction, faithful in prayer. Share with the Lord's people who are in need. Practice hospitality.

ROMANS 12:9-13 NIV

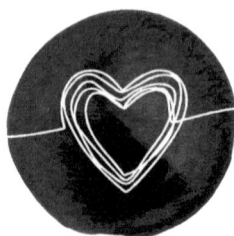

— Father's Heart —

Life is a gift—

One not meant to be about you alone, My child—not because you aren't important, but because I know how much you flourish when in community with others. I designed you this way, and it's beautiful to see your heart wired with perfect intricacy for village life.

Are you heavy-hearted, weary or tired of the depths you now walk?

One thing that can help is taking a peek outside your own walls. Look up and beyond the constant pressure of your current season.

This is no mere mistake; I created you for kinship—each pouring into one another in healthy, selfless loving acts of kindness.

One lifts another, and when one is lowly, I bring another to uplift them.

Even if no one is willing, I will show up Myself for them!

I invite you into this place of give and receive as led by My heart. Do you want adventure? You

*want more in life? You want to feel as though
you are not alone in all you are and do?*

Time to connect. Time to rise above your situation and pour.

*Don't worry; you won't be doing this from your
resource and energy alone; I will provide all
that you need. Lo and behold, you'll find yourself
with over and above what you give out.*

*My currency makes no human sense, and you're
realising I do not work as the world works—this makes
Me laugh out loud! I did not create you only to look
inside yourself, but to the needs of those around you.*

I created you to be communal and relational, My child.

*When you find yourself only focusing on the
things happening within you and to you.
Where am I? Where are you looking?*

*Circumstances will look to distract you from what I
want for you. They will try and take your eyes from Me,
and instead focus on the things that bring you down,
loading heavy weights upon you that obscure hope.*

Life feels harder than it needs to be in this place.

*My words and ways are the ones that will bring
life. They will encourage, lighten, and brighten
your days, and the days of those around you.*

*When My children choose to look to others it
brings Me great joy, as does their loving one
another out of My strength and abundance.*

*My loving plans long to lift your eyes from what you
see, what you feel or what you humanly know, moving*

them toward Me. As your focus shifts, you see beyond your current circumstance. It's often out of your weakness when I can work with you. Investing and bringing life to someone else brings much to others, but also to you as you exchange heaviness for hope.

This idea of exchange is not a new concept, but one that bears My very heartbeat to you—if you'll choose to see.

If you are in a lowly place, ask Me to highlight someone for you. As you pray, I will lift and bring life to the both of you.

Kind words are like honey, sweet to the
soul and healthy for the body.

PROVERBS 16:24 NLT

And do not forget to do good and to share with others, for with such sacrifices God is pleased.

HEBREWS 13:16 NIV

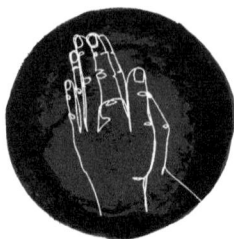

— Prayer —

Creative, generous, and loving God,

I know there have been times where I've been so wrapped up in my own world and its problems, that it's become bigger than it needs to be.

Thank You that You have often brought someone from outside my inner world, to speak Your words, tend, comfort or give to.

I have LOVED these God adventures.

Living my own life, unaffected and unaware of those around me is quite easy, but You have adventures all around, ready to be leapt into.

Lord, whatever You put on my heart today, I will do.

If You ask me to talk with a stranger, then I will.

If You ask me to give something, I will give it.

If You ask me to do something that reflects Your heart of love, I will do it.

Help me to go into the day, keeping an eye out for Your prompts — those times where You highlight people and opportunities to partner with You.

Thank You, precious Father, for it all.

Amen.

XXXXX

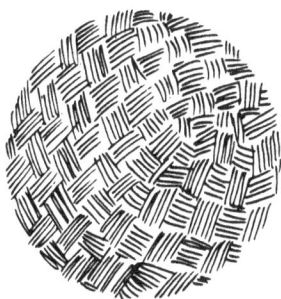

Chapter Ten

SOUND TEACHING

For I give you sound teaching;
do not abandon my instruction.

PROVERBS 4:2 NASB

Holding fast the faithful word which is in accordance with the teaching, so that he will be able to both exhort in sound doctrine and to refute those who contradict.

TITUS 1:9 NASB 1995

had always loved shopping with Holy Spirit.

He often drew my eye to something "random," and not long after, I'd realise why He had me purchase it. I hadn't realised He was leading me, but it was always fun to see the hows and whys unfold.

These light, joyous shopping experiences were, of course, before the health crisis began. Shopping had not been in my recent list of activities.

Night times had become a time of dread. Sleep often evading me.

Just walking into the bedroom at night-time, I would sweat, as panic set in.

Night times meant refreshing sleep for everyone around me; but for me, this was not the case. Intense fear and the sense of being alone gripped my insides and twisted painfully.

As I lay there, waiting for sleep to come, intensity and fear sought to overcome me instead.

My lids refused to remain closed, as every sound caused my nervous system to jump.

Every organ internally moving and processing the day that had preceded this moment in time.

What's this? What does that pain mean?

My body would ping and pang, sometimes waking me from the rare snippets of sleep.

This isn't sustainable.

How long can a person live without good sleep? Will it ever get better, Lord?

I'd heard people mention dark nights of the soul. Every night for months, it had become this for me. The atmosphere seemed to weigh into the terror I felt each night.

I prayed, declared, and did everything I humanly could to stop this living nightmare, but to no avail.

As the sun fell from the sky and the moon rose, a horrible sensation gripped my being, and nothing seemed to be able to alleviate it. As soon as I began my night-time routine, a wash of anxiety would come over me, and humanly I couldn't shake it.

Just when I felt I couldn't do one more night like this, I felt Holy Spirit bring a picture to my mind.

Remember your CD pile.

I saw a picture of a stack of compact discs. I saw the spines of each one, sitting like a stack of books on a shelf.

One, in particular, seemed to be highlighted, as it leapt out to me.

It looked appealing, interesting.

The Lord's Prayer Teaching Series.

The pastors at church had taught a series six months ago on this subject.

It was solid, healthy teaching, and when it was offered as a take-home teaching series, that same shopping Holy Spirit prompt zipped into my heart.

It had come home with us on the Sunday, and I'd put it on our bookshelf. And there it had sat on my shelf these past months—untouched, unopened, and unlistened to.

Now is the time to have a listen, beloved.

Willing to try anything, as the clock hit 8 p.m., my trembling hands carefully placed the silver disc into the player.

JUST WHEN I FELT I COULDN'T DO ONE MORE NIGHT LIKE THIS, I FELT HOLY SPIRIT BRING A PICTURE TO MY MIND.

I snuggled under the covers, endeavouring to settle my internal buzzing. Deep-breathing exercises calmed me enough to enable me to focus on the words which swam across the room to my ears.

Fifteen minutes passed by.

As the teaching was released into the atmosphere of our bedroom, my nervous system settled.

This is different. I feel at ease and peaceful.

I've not felt this for months. My body is settling to traditionally normal rhythms.

"What is this, Lord?"

As if my body systems were being sung a lullaby, they were soothed by the reassuring truth of God's Word being spoken.

I felt God working in me through the words — as something shifted in the surrounding atmosphere. As if the darkness was being replaced with light, our bedroom felt fresher and lighter. The air felt different and more readily inhaled.

Oh, Lord, this is wonderful.

The teaching was sound…solid. No human opinions, just brilliant Bible teaching. How my heart had missed this kind of investment over the past months.

Night times are going to look a whole lot different as I listen to stuff like this!

Each night I would turn on the series.

The moment I turned it on, peace would tangibly enter within moments, like a welcome friend come to visit, bringing a blanket and hugs.

> NIGHT TIMES ARE GOING TO LOOK A WHOLE LOT DIFFERENT AS I LISTEN TO STUFF LIKE THIS!

The teaching was on the Lord's prayer (Matthew 6:9-13). I usually only made it through the first couple of sessions. Ken's voice was so calming, and the teaching was so pure that it seemed to wash away all heaviness.

The fear and sense of darkness happened occasionally, but more nights than not, God used this method as a key to enter His peace.

Following these months of poor sleep, I shared with Ken the impact the teaching had made in my life. It's not often a pastor would be pleased to hear their teaching put someone to sleep, but thankfully Ken found it humorous.

In pointing out these things to the brethren, you will be a good servant of Christ Jesus, constantly nourished on the words of the faith and of the sound doctrine which you have been following.

1 TIMOTHY 4:6 NASB 1995

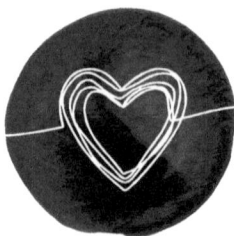

— Father's Heart —

I have placed before you an abundance of food—teaching that would feed the entire world for 1000 years.

I partner with My children to speak life into your situation through this rich feast.

Walk alongside Me and ask where to begin.

I will place the keys in your palm, so all you need is to put the key in the lock and turn it.

Do you need clarity?

Do you need peace?

Do you need next steps and instruction?

Do you need hope in your current season?

Are you lacking something, but don't know what?

Getting back to My foundations, My solid teaching is good for your health, body, soul and mind.

Feed on the things of My heart, and you'll find yourself never wanting.

*The world has so much to offer, and at
times it can be overwhelming.*

*I take your hand and gently lead you to the
things that count. Those teachings which will
speak right to the heart of the matter.*

I long for you to grasp My heartbeat and love for you.

*My Spirit will guide you to the best teaching
for your circumstance which will help you
to step out in My freedom once more.*

*There is a smorgasbord of teaching before you, and this can
become overwhelming at times. As you walk closely with
Me, you'll become familiar with My wisdom and truth.*

Ask Me to protect your heart from that which is not of Me.

*Then ask Me to allow the things that your body, mind, soul,
emotions, and spirit need to soak in and consume heartily.*

*A message given by Me through a teacher can change
your circumstance and the world around you.*

*My inspired teaching draws the heart
towards Me and speaks with authority, truth,
and always with love at its core.*

*Take, eat of the good food I have placed before you.
Then go into the world where I have placed you and
let My words inspire and empower you to do good
works, to speak life and to walk in My freedom.*

*Do this that others may see and acknowledge
Me, that they will turn and thank Me for you
and the things you have done in My name.*

SOUND TEACHING

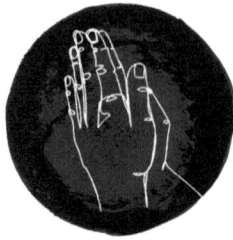

— Prayer —

Father of all sound teaching,

Lord, I want to be firmly planted in Your truth.

Keep the eyes of my heart open and attuned to the things of You.

*Continue to give me wisdom and discernment
to know whether something is of You.*

Please bring the right teaching to me at the right time.

Please let my heart listen to and hear Your words.

Let me never esteem the teacher more than the teaching.

*Bless those who choose the often-challenging road of being
a voice of influence for You here on earth. Bless their
relationships with You, with their spouse and their family.*

*Lead me, Father. Guide me to where You want me to
be and who You want me to listen to or read from.*

*Show me the ones who will preach
You, both in Spirit and in truth.*

Amen.

XXXXX

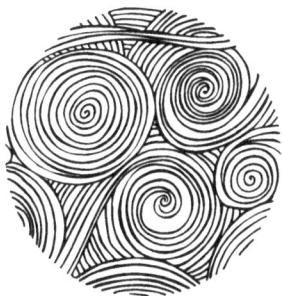

Chapter Eleven

THE WORD

In the beginning was the Word, and the
Word was with God, and the Word was God.

JOHN 1:1 NKJV

All Scripture is God-breathed and is useful for teaching, rebuking, correcting and training in righteousness, so that the servant of God may be thoroughly equipped for every good work.

2 TIMOTHY 3:16-17 NIV

Finally, our new home was built, and moving day was within reach.

The idea of selling our current home brought with it a sense of dread and anxiety.

Where is this coming from, Father?

It was March 4, 2014, and my heart was making connections with the long, stressful sale of our previous home.

Ugh, that was a horrible time. What if it's the same?

I can't do that again, Lord. I don't want to deal with real-estate agents and open days. Argh, it was a loooong five months of selling.

Our agent had proved to be manipulative and dishonorable, which brought a LOT of additional drama to our already stressful situation.

The worry tornado swirled in my heart, as I wrestled with old memories and new situations.

Realisation HIT!

I have no control over what happens.

Be still; sit with Me, My beloved. Tell me all about your worries and fears. I am with You. I will help you work it out.

I sat down to try and make sense of it with God.

Journaling all my worries until my hand grew weary from writing the list of things I could not control, my writing highlighted three main concerns.

1. The timeline. Would it take as long, and if so, how would I cope?

2. The people. What if the real-estate agent did the same thing? Are we safe?

3. The future. Will we actually get onto the land and into our new home?

And here I was, March 4, 2014, in the same position of selling our home in order to finally moved to the block God had highlighted all those years before.

Continue reading the Word, My child. Pick up from where you finished reading yesterday: Psalm 37.

As I read, my mouth dropped to the floor, my eyes grew round like dinner plates, and my hands began to shake with an adrenaline surge.

"Be still before the Lord and wait patiently for him; do not fret when people succeed in their ways, when they carry out their wicked schemes. Refrain from anger and turn from

> JOURNALING ALL
> MY WORRIES
> UNTIL MY HAND
> GREW WEARY
> FROM WRITING
> THE LIST OF
> THINGS I COULD
> NOT CONTROL,
> MY WRITING
> HIGHLIGHTED
> THREE MAIN
> CONCERNS.

wrath; do not fret — it leads only to evil. For evil men will be destroyed, but those who hope in the Lord will inherit the land." Psalm 37: 7-9

The words leapt off the page towards me, piercing my heart afresh.

Oh, Lord! Thank You! Whatever happens, You have said we will inherit the land. You have told me not to worry; I need only be still before You. Thank You!

I sat a while, meditating on how this passage might be practically applied.

As I sat there, He brought to mind a testimony of a house-selling time where God had also been so faithful. I turned to the passage.

"'I saw the Lord always before me.
　　Because he is at my right hand,
　　I will not be shaken.
　Therefore my heart is glad and my tongue rejoices;
　　my body also will rest in hope,
because you will not abandon me to the realm of the dead,
　　you will not let your holy one see decay.
You have made known to me the paths of life;
　　you will fill me with joy in your presence.
　　　　Acts 2:25-28 NIV

Immediately I was transported to the morning I had written those words years before the house was finally sold to the people who were meant for it all along. I was in tears, crying out to God, walking through this horrible mystery time, questioning everything. I had reached the end of myself, and He'd prompted my heart to choose not to leave my chair until I had heard from Him, through His word.

Take a closer look, My child. His warm smile spreading across His lips as He spoke these words to me.

THE WORD

Intrigued, I looked again and felt pulled to the tiny handwritten notes in the border of my Bible, beside the highlighted Acts 2:25-28. You could've knocked me over with a feather as I read the following:

"23 July 2000. House selling…general stress."

and then beneath it,

"23 July 2010. House selling. Weird… Lord, I leave this in Your hands from this day forth. You have gone before us on this journey, and we will not be shaken. In Jesus' powerful name, Amen."

It was the exact passage that I had read all those years before.

It was the same encouragement from Him for the same circumstance we had walked through 10 years prior — a reminder of what God had done all those years ago.

Miraculously, He had brought me to the same verse ten years to the day since I had written the testimony in the margin!

TAKE A CLOSER LOOK, MY CHILD. HIS WARM SMILE SPREADING ACROSS HIS LIPS AS HE SPOKE THESE WORDS TO ME.

Same situation.

Same problem.

Same verse.

Same promise.

I don't think I had read that passage in between the two sales.

You came through then, why not now!?

Freshly assured of a redemptive outcome.

I trust You Lord with this sale. I will not worry or fear any more about it with Your help.

Our home sold within the week, a short settlement and the real estate agent was greatly blessed by seeing what God did in the sale.

His Word proved true — yet again.

Why do I ever doubt it?

For the word of God is alive and active. Sharper than any two-edged sword, it penetrates even to dividing soul and spirit, joints and marrow; it judges the thoughts and the attitudes of the heart.

HEBREWS 4:12 NIV

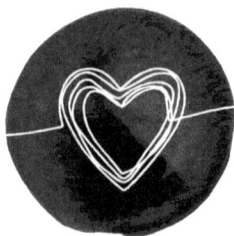

— Father's Heart —

My Word is My bond.

It is My promise to you that you are never alone.

It holds personal life promises,
made just for your time and season.

It holds the ultimate story of hope and forgiveness.

It gives you reason and purpose.

I set out My guidelines to live well and with fullness of joy.

I have created you to be a part of My Word.

You are an integral part of My story.

You have a choice, My child, to be a part of My story or
not; this is free will. I will not force this upon you.

Rest before Me and ask Me to show you where to begin.

Then read, rest and listen. Being aware of Me can help, but even
if you don't "feel" Me, keep reading until My Spirit highlights a
word or a passage. This is where you can stop and let it soak in.

Ask my Holy Spirit to reveal the truth of what you are reading.

Ask me how it relates to you right now.

Reading while in a hurried space can leave My Word feeling lifeless and without power. You've tried that many times before; let's try something better for your design.

Come worship and rest before Me; then My presence will make the Word come alive in you.

It is always living, but you need to be active in it to come alive!

When this happens, My Word will leap off the page and speak to your exact situation.

Feed yourself by being in My Word. It was written just for you.

I give you every reason to know that you are loved and valued.

I know you so well, My child, and I want the best for you.

Come to Me and My Word often. I will speak to you. I will encourage you.

I will instruct you to eat from the buffets of richness before your enemies!

My Word will guide you, teach and uplift you.

I will tell you what to do and when. Mysteries will be solved, confusion made clear and the way ahead clarified as you learn to trust Me, asking questions and then where to find the answers.

My Spirit will prompt you with answers or guide you where to begin.

Explore My Word, dwell in it, let it infiltrate your heart and the very best of Me will shine through you.

THE WORD

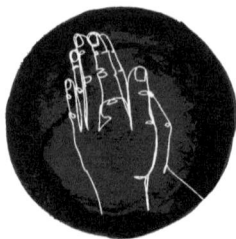

— *Prayer* —

O Lord,

Thank You for Your Son, Jesus, Who is the Word.

You come to life through Your Word and in my heart.

*Thank You for giving us all that we
will ever need for flourishing.*

I love that You know who I am and what I need.

Help me to hear Your voice clearly through Your living Word.

*Father, I love it when Your Word comes alive in
me; please remove anything that hinders this.*

I love it when we meet, and You show me the paths of life.

*Please continue to reveal more of what I need through
Your Word, so I can be salt and light to those around me.*

*Tend to my heart and show me great and
hidden things that I didn't know before.*

My future is sure and secure in You.

Thank You, precious Father. I love You and Your Word so much.

XXXXX

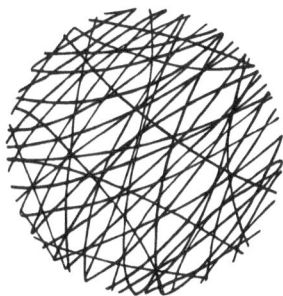

Chapter Twelve

VISIONS

And the Spirit lifted me up and brought me in a vision
by the Spirit of God to the exiles in Chaldea. So the
vision that I had seen left me. Then I told the exiles
all the things that the LORD had shown me.

EZEKIEL 11:24-25 NASB 1995

On the next day, as they were on their way and approaching the city, Peter went up on the housetop about the sixth hour to pray. But he became hungry and was desiring to eat; but while they were making preparations, he fell into a trance; and he saw the sky opened up, and an object like a great sheet coming down, lowered by four corners to the ground.

ACTS 10:9-11 NASB 1995

Sitting in my favourite thinking chair. Its thick beige material has large, funky brown leaves scattered across the textured fabric. I loved settling down into it, my arms taking hold of the wide timber arms, lifting my feet onto the matching ottoman.

I feel safe, secure, ready to meet Father.

This chair had been my soaking chair. My grieving chair. My revelation chair. My healing chair.

Faced towards the lofty gum trees which spread across the horizon, this was an unrushed place, my place of rest with Him.

The week had been one of rush and bustle, hinting at years of the former me. It seemed the more healed I became, the more that was required of me.

I'd set this time apart to spend time with God once again.

THIS CHAIR HAD BEEN MY SOAKING CHAIR. MY GRIEVING CHAIR. MY REVELATION CHAIR. MY HEALING CHAIR.

Not the fast quiet time on my way to elsewhere — but an agenda-less morning for Him and me.

I miss You, Lord.

I'm sorry for buying into busyness. I feel pulled in every direction, and yet the activity isn't satisfying. It leaves me depleted and alone.

Why?

I've been giving out to others for weeks, and my bucket is depleted to drops.

As stores ran dry and in desperate need of refreshment, I sat; my heart rested with Him.

No thinking or moving.

Simply being. Set apart time to be with the source of my strength and refreshment.

Without warning, a scene unfolded before my eyes — as real as if it was in the room with me. A living picture.

Or am I in it? I'm not sure.

A country scene.

A walkable hill with a quaint little cottage perched at its peak.

Spiraling smoke weaved its way leisurely out of the chimney, suggesting a fire had been lit.

Jesus appeared beside me, and we walked hand in hand towards the cottage.

All was at ease.

My heart enjoying the easy, unhurried pace of Jesus in this place.

No questions or thinking about my long to-do list. He and I were simply taking a gentle stroll up a hill.

What delight!

Arriving at the cottage and I noted the heavy, handcrafted door was wide open, welcoming us in.

At this point I felt a little unsure about going inside, but Jesus ushered me in with a reassuring smile.

Taking my first step inside, I landed on the rustic bluestone block floor. My eyes tracked the lines of the mortar between the blocks eventually leading to the fireplace.

JESUS APPEARED BESIDE ME, AND WE WALKED HAND IN HAND TOWARDS THE COTTAGE.

The comforting flames danced and flickered about. A generous, high-backed chair sat before the warming fire. In the chair sat Father God.

My heart skipped a beat as I saw Him, His hands outstretched motioning for me to come closer.

Back in my brown-leaf chair, I felt myself in both places. Whether my eyes were open or closed, I could see and sense the vision He was giving me. Instinctively I knew that I could choose to remain with Him in it or leave it.

How is this happening?

But the thought disappeared as quickly as it came.

I want to be with You, Father.

I neared His chair, feeling more at ease than I'd felt my entire life.

So much communicated in that wordless moment.

Dwelling. No rush, no scurry; but communing.

The room was cosy comfort and felt like home, the moment I entered. The firelight seemed to fill the room as much as was needed. The flickering illuminating Him, the focus of this inviting room.

VISIONS

This is my kind of place.

I could live here, Father. It's beautiful.

Father motioned with His large hand, **"Have you seen my walls, My beloved?"**

The light crept to the outer edges of the room, revealing walls which reached all the way up to the sky.

Each wall littered from top to bottom with photo frames. A mix of empty and filled ones.

In awe of how it could be such an intimate space, when the walls seemed to have no end, I looked back at Father, amazed.

He grinned with a knowing kind of look, waiting for me to glance at the walls. Upon closer inspection, I realised the photos in the frames were of me.

FATHER MOTIONED WITH HIS LARGE HAND, "HAVE YOU SEEN MY WALLS, MY BELOVED?"

"Lord, these are photos from my life."

"Yes, My child. I love to take photos of the things no one else notices."

My jaw dropped, deeply moved by His words.

He sees me.

He notices every little thing.

He loves me that much.

As lover of photography and a self-confessed snap-happy parent, this really resonated.

Wow....

The photos were surprising and didn't highlight those upfront moments of my life. Rather, the times when I had stopped and talked with people on the street. Listened to and spoken kindly to sales assistants. Those times I had been prompted to give secret gifts or pour love into others. The photos depicted those moments where my heart was moved by Him.

Those times of gentle obedience.

Thrilled. Humbled.

God had noticed! He had noticed all those times.

He took pictures of them; He treasured them.

The empty frames…these frames are the things yet to come.

I noticed how many empty frames there were. In my earthly lifetime, I'd barely touched the surface of all the frames yet to come.

Oh, Lord, thank You!

I became aware of wide arms my hands were resting upon. Reaching down to my trusty box of tissues, mopping the tears which had inadvertently been pouring from my eyes.

What an encouragement!

This filled me with hope and excitement for the future.

What a gift! What a gift! At this time, when I found any physical exertion difficult and feared at times whether I had any worth or future at all, this encouragement was pure gold!

I didn't understand logically what had just happened, but it drew me closer to His heart, revealing a place of safety, love, and revelation with Him.

I hadn't done anything special to bring it about, but God knew how He wanted to communicate, and today, it was through a treasured vision — a vision which would continue to encourage me for years to come.

After these things the word of the LORD came to
Abram in a vision, saying, "Do not fear, Abram, I am
a shield to you; your reward shall be very great."

GENESIS 15:1 NASB 1995

Boasting is necessary, though it is not profitable; but I
will go on to visions and revelations of the Lord. I know
a man in Christ who fourteen years ago — whether in the
body I do not know, or out of the body I do not know, God
knows — such a man was caught up to the third heaven.

2 CORINTHIANS 12:1-4 NASB 1995

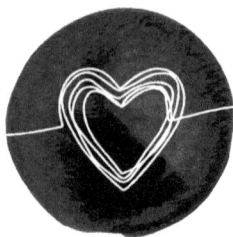

— Father's Heart —

*As you connect with and trust Me, I will show you
great and inexplicable things. I long to show you
more, but you are not quite ready for that, My child.*

*Come and trust Me to show and tell you whatever
you need for that moment and beyond.*

I give visions for specific purposes.

*I use them as keys to speak to you and show you something
you need to see, to experience. I long to reveal more
of My heart to you — sometimes this will be through
the gift of pictures or moving interactive visions.*

*Trust Me with whatever and however
I wish to speak with you.*

Be open to new lines of communication, My child.

*Things you could not even imagine, but as you know
Me, you can trust Me, child. I will not lead you astray.*

*Test these things that you receive, and if they do
not fit with My nature and word, let them go.*

*If they do align with Who I am and My
Word, then embrace them. I will show you
wonderful truths through them.*

*Like dreams, pictures and any way I speak to you, visions
instruct, teach, reveal, encourage, heal and inspire and
more. They will ultimately draw you closer to Me, building
our intimacy and helping to write our together story.*

*Expect the unexpected. Develop an awareness of Me
desiring connection and intimacy—with Who I
am as our focus. Instead of what I do, or can bring
for you, above all else, desire Me, beloved.*

*Sometimes you might find yourself looking at the journey
of others, wishing you had this gift or that encounter.*

*Do not be disappointed about how I show
Myself to you, or how I speak to you.*

*I know you best and know there are times you have
desired something other than what I am giving you.*

*Trust Me with how I reveal Myself, and you
will be in the safest hands—Mine.*

*I love you dearly, My precious child. There
is much adventure ahead, so hang on to Me
tightly; let our adventures begin.*

VISIONS

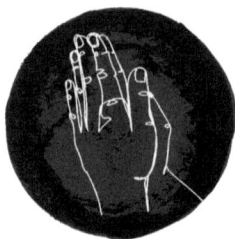

— *Prayer* —

Precious Father,

You are a creative and wonderful God.

I marvel at Who You are and what You do in my world.

I don't always understand or know the context of what You bring to me, but I am confident that You will reveal it at exactly the right time.

Help my eyes to always see what You have put right in front of me, Father.

I don't wish to be closed to the things of You.

Keep my heart soft, Holy Spirit. Allow me to be responsive to Your promptings and encouragements.

Help me to remain secure in our relationship and receptive to how and when You wish to speak.

Allow the security I have in You to ground me.

I have confidence in what You have for me.

Develop a contentment in me to enjoy the journey as I encounter You in the ways You know I need; and if that is receiving a vision from You, I am open, Lord.

In Jesus' name,
Amen.

XXXXX

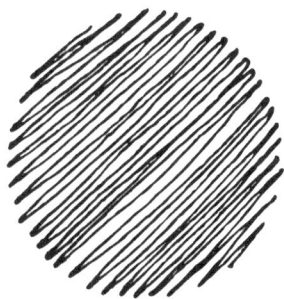

Chapter Thirteen

DREAMS

To these four young men God gave knowledge and understanding of all kinds of literature and learning. And Daniel could understand visions and dreams of all kinds.

DANIEL 1:17 NIV

"And it shall come to pass afterward, that I will pour out my Spirit on all flesh; your sons and your daughters shall prophesy, your old men shall dream dreams, and your young men shall see visions."

JOEL 2:28 ESV

I'm amazed at how You work, Lord!

This past year had been one of the richest years of my life so far.

As I'd finished up my study year, I felt a little lost, as my community of learners went their separate ways.

It's hard to have a camp-like experience with a group, so tight knit and then have to move into a new season.

DO YOU SEE WHAT I HAVE ALREADY GIVEN YOU?

What does this season hold, Lord?

My body is still recovering from the intensity of having pushed it beyond its limits — now what?

Do you see what I have already given you?

Do you remember your group of prophetic dreamers?

They are where I want you to invest time this year.

Start, take the next step, and the rest will follow. It's going to be good.

My heart leapt at the idea of already having a community online to whom I felt drawn. Knowing nothing about dreaming with God, but constantly dreaming at night times, it seemed a great fit for my heart.

The fact that there was a prophetic leaning towards the group's vision, was a bonus!

Erica was attending Bethel Church in Redding and had begun a prophetic dreamers' group where we would ask God for interpretations for people. Only as I joined this group did dreaming become HUGE in my life.

I was greatly humbled to be asked to join the small team of interpreters, and they became my online church family. Over the course of the year, we became so close, and as we poured out what God revealed, people were blessed. The Facebook group grew from hundreds to at last count 16000. Erica's dream for a healthy, encouraging, equipping dream community was a reality.

Erica had been obedient in starting the group—drawing together a passionate group of people who asked God for interpretations for others in dreams and working together as a community.

As the year progressed, we became closer, actually living out what my heart has always felt church could be—intimate, vulnerable, encouraging, regularly communicating, sharing revelations and God insights.

I felt as if I had been on the top of a wave for most of the year. Surfing into shore, the wind in my hair, droplets of water refreshing me.

This is what I was destined to do.

I LOVE dreams and learning about what You would say through them, Lord! Thank You.

I hadn't always remembered my dreams.

Only when Erica was given some insight about blockers to dreaming with God that I took some action.

"Lord, if there is anything I or others have said or done that is stopping me from attuning to You through dreams, I'm sorry. Please forgive me. Cleanse the lines of communication between You and me, make my night times about listening to You.

I give You my dreams, my nights and any sleep that I have. Feel free to use these nine hours as You like."

THIS IS WHAT I WAS DESTINED TO DO.

The moment I prayed this prayer, I felt a lightness enter my heart and mind. The frustration I used to feel at not being able to fall asleep, tossing and turning for hours on end; waking in the middle of the night for hours, lying there, not knowing what to think or do….now I had an assignment. A purpose for this time!

"Lord, You are King of my night times and my dreams, I ask You to protect my family and me as we sleep. Surround us with Your heavenly angels, so that all the wakeful parts of me will attune to You, and the rest will rest in Your presence."

To offer my night times to God seemed a simple thing. I didn't expect anything much to happen. But from that moment, I began dreaming every single night.

Lord, I can't remember all that You're showing and telling me. I don't want to miss it.

I want you to put a journal beside your bed, My child. You will lie down and dream in peace with Me. I will prompt you with words, pictures and stories that you'll be able to note down the main things. In the morning I'll connect the dots with you.

DREAMS

And this is what began to happen.

Along with my prophetic dreaming group, the area of dreams began to unfold and explode in my world.

Processing dreams.

Healing dreams.

Instructional dreams.

Encouragement dreams.

Strategic dreams.

Symbolic dreams.

Revelationary dreams.

Action dreams.

Adventurous dreams.

Intimacy with the Father dreams and so many more.

If I had problems in everyday life, God would often use my night times — those times when it was only Him and me in the quiet — to respond.

If others had issues, if some needed intercession, encouragement, clarity, He was faithful in FULL.

To write all the things that dreams can be would fill libraries of books. (See appendix 1 for some specific testimonies.)

But the power of dreaming with God, connecting with others who shared my heart in this season, proved life-changing and a true gift.

Thank You, Lord!

Now when they had departed, behold, an angel of the Lord appeared to Joseph in a dream and said, "Rise, take the child and his mother, and flee to Egypt, and remain there until I tell you, for Herod is about to search for the child, to destroy him."

MATTHEW 2:13 ESV

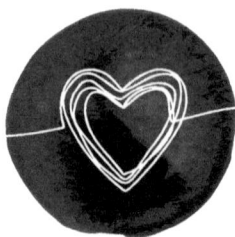

— Father's Heart —

As your body and mind rest at night, it is an ideal time for Me to speak life into your tired body.

I love to watch over you as you sleep. Give Me all the cares of your day before you go to sleep, My child. Then snuggle up and rest in Me.

As you become aware of My presence around you, welcome Me into your dreams and find rest in Me.

The days seems long at times, and your nights have been a struggle too. It's time for Me to reclaim the night for you—if you will allow Me.

Trust Me to protect you as you sleep.

As your body begins to rest and your mind follows, thank Me for being with you and then hand over your sleep time to Me.

During these times I love to pour refreshment into you.

During these times I speak to you of things to come.

During these times I give you ideas to act upon.

*I love to give you answers during this
time because you are finally still.*

*One way I speak to you is through dreams. I have always
done this. I love to show you My heartbeat and reveal
more about Myself during this special time together.*

*I will invest peace into you physically during this time, so
that you can step into whatever needs peace when you wake.*

*I enjoy showing you scenes of life during your dreaming.
Some will be practical and obvious. Others will be
symbolic, requiring you to ask Me for more clarity when
you wake. Others will be prophetic details for the future.*

*In fact, sometimes when you might feel like you
have lived something before as it is happening, I
had already given you a dream about it.*

*I will also give you answers to questions that have been
troubling you. I am giving you a gift in your dreams.*

*Trust Me with your dream life and begin to take notice
of what you go to sleep with and wake up with.*

*These ideas can be powerful truths
that bless both you and others.*

*Listen to My instruction and ask Me if you don't understand.
I will reveal all, at the right time, as you seek Me.*

*I am excited to think that you might invite My Spirit
to meet with you as you sleep, providing Me with eight
hours of uninterrupted listening time, my child. I
love it when I have your full attention and heart.*

DREAMS

*As you hand these times over to Me, trust Me to
bring you goodness every step of the way.*

*Because I love you, and I want the
absolute best for you, My beloved."*

If you lie down, you will not be afraid; when
you lie down, your sleep will be sweet.

PROVERBS 3:24 ESV

"When there is a prophet among you, I, the LORD, reveal myself to them in visions, I speak to them in dreams."

NUMBERS 12:6 NIV

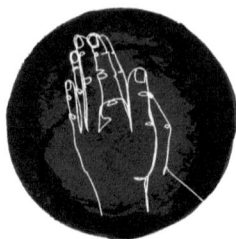

— Prayer —

O Heavenly Father,

Thank You for enabling us to experience dreams.

*You LOVE to give good gifts to Your kids; please
help me be willing and open to receive these.*

I love it when You connect with me through my dreams.

Thank You that this is another way for You to create and restore.

*Father, please remind me to give You complete
control over my life, especially as I sleep.*

I trust You to lead me to watering holes of refreshment in my dreams.

Please use my night times for Your purposes.

*I hand over my heart, mind, emotions, body, all that
is asleep and awake to You during these times.*

Father, if You wish to reveal something to me, please reveal it.

If You wish to provide answers to questions I have, please do this too.

*If You wish to bring messages of encouragement
for others, bring those too.*

I love Your ways, precious Father.

Amen.

XXXXX

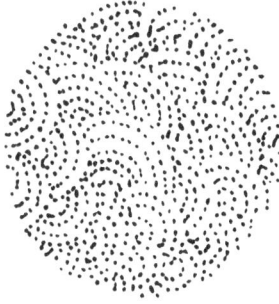

Chapter Fourteen

THANKFULNESS

But I will sacrifice to You with the voice of thanksgiving....

JONAH 2:9A NASB 1995

I will bless the LORD at all times; his praise
shall continually be in my mouth.

PSALM 34:1 ESV

Ugh, Lord, I feel terrible. Stop the world, I want to get off!

I need a holiday, Lord, a slower pace, less life clutter and busyness.

Business, family, friends, church and personal stress hills were melding together and becoming quite a mountain.

It seemed one of those seasons where everyone was going through heavy.

My phone pinged every hour—alerting me to messages of people needing prayer, help or just to vent.

I've had enough, Lord!

I turned my phone on silent to try and keep myself from tipping into overwhelm.

Focus on breathing…no change.

Prayed, claimed and declared…but my body systems continued to race and zaps of nerve pain shocked me out of sweet spaces.

Even creating with art supplies, I was unable to focus enough to enjoy the process.

My old faithfuls weren't working today.

My internals raced and ran and pinged and panged. Today was a day where they couldn't be ignored.

Entering the bathroom to wash my face and brush my teeth, I noted the ghostly pale face in the mirror before me. I looked as tired as I felt inside.

No makeup, raw, headachy and sore all over. *This is the worst I've felt in a looooong time.*

Is there anything I can do to help this, Lord? I don't want to crash. Can I stop it somehow?

THANKFEST — ONE LINER THANKFUL DECLARATIONS.

Thank Me.

Huh? How? Anything specific?

My brain didn't seem to be able to connect with my heart too well today.

Remember what you did with your kids on the way to school. It's time to revisit it.

I recalled a God prompt from years ago — a fun little activity that God dropped into my spirit one morning when the kids were bickering and sibling rivalry was rife.

I'd had enough then too....and before I knew it, I demanded that we all settle down and suggested we have a "thankfest." That phrase left my lips before I had a plan about what that might mean.

Thank You, Lord.

The kids stopped in their tracks, ceased the fighting from the backseat and collectively asked that key question, "What's a thankfest?"

"We are only a few minutes from school. Let's see if we can thank God for anything that comes to mind all the way to school."

They thought this was a great idea! And I breathed a sigh of relief that the bickering had subsided.

Thankfest—one liner thankful declarations.

Over time it morphed, and we mixed it up to keep it interesting.

We'd set a challenge to see if we could give thanks for set times, topics and people. Sometimes we'd just have thankfest unlimited—where we could thank God for anything.

We always found that by the end of the car trip, we had had some fun and had started our days well. The atmosphere in the car had lifted considerably, and we had forgotten the tension only moments before.

What've I got to lose, today—this challenging day? It's worth a go.

"Thank You, God, for life. Thank You for my family. For having food available. For a roof over our heads."

I found myself covering the essentials—the easy and the seen. When I couldn't think of another tangible thing, I took stock…feeling a little better for having thanked God for these things.

I then turned to some ouchy areas—the business, other people's problems, the areas that were drawing from my energy stores—the very things I felt very "unthankful" for.

Please help me reframe these thankfully, Lord.

"Thank You, God, for all the work. Thank You for those people who pay quickly. Thank You for those who haven't yet, and that You care about them too.

Bless their business, so that they can pay their bills.

God, thank You for the privilege of having time for people. Thank You for being trustworthy and allowing others to share with me their hearts.

Thank You that You have ways for me to balance my boundaries and navigate this in healthier ways.

Thank You that You aren't overwhelmed by all that is around You. Thank You that I don't have to care more about others' problems than they do. Thank You that I can hand these burdens over to You quickly so they don't become weights around my neck."

Woah…..He's giving me strategies through the thanks, coming from His heart through my own mouth.

"Thank You, God. Oh, thank You, God."

AS I THANKED GOD, THE HEAD PRESSURE LESSENED.

Hope was being restored…like being in the desert with an empty bucket and having cool, refreshing water poured in and filled back up. The air seemed to be physically returning to my lungs as I took a satisfying deep breath, the vagus nerve settled and blessed digestion, blood pressure and lung ease.

"Thank You, Lord!"

The energy in my near overstimulated nervous system that had been buzzing just moments before, had now subsided. The headache remained.

I felt to thank God for those things that He had promised me—those things that were yet to be fully realised.

"God, I thank You for my health. I thank You that this headache will go because it doesn't belong in heaven. Thank You that I have

Your full assurance of healing. Thank You that my body is a blessing to me. Thank You for giving me a body that serves me so well. Thank You for it all."

As I thanked God, the head pressure lessened.

I spent the rest of the afternoon continuing to thank God for whatever came to mind. I rested. I hydrated.

God, how can I bless my body today?

Ideas would come to mind.

I'd follow through with what He showed me to do.

By the end of the day, as I washed my hands at the sink, I caught another glimpse of my face in the mirror…it had colour and life again in it. The worry lines had dissipated—less weary. In fact, I looked as though I'd been at the beach and got a bit of a suntan, but of course, I hadn't.

How do You do that, Lord?

How do You turn a rotten morning into a redemptive day? From overwhelmed systems to light and free? You are amazing!

Thankfulness is a weapon—not a weakness, daughter.

Giving thanks is a mover and a shaker for the things that would come at you.

Give thanks often.

Give thanks when you feel like it, but better still, even when you don't. Especially when you don't. You'll find yourself better off for having given thanks in these times.

> THANKFULNESS IS A WEAPON — NOT A WEAKNESS, DAUGHTER.

THANKFULNESS

Are you afflicted, tired, worn out, or overwhelmed? My beloved, these are the times to remember Me. Remember My promises.

Declare My goodness and truth.

As you speak out thanks, you will discover an oasis in the desert and a wellspring of life. Speak life. Release thanks. Praise Me always, and I say again give thanks.

I bowed my head, humbled by all that He had done.

"Thank You, Lord! Help me to remember to do this especially when things feel beyond me. You are soooooo GOOD."

O give thanks to the LORD, for He is GOOD;
for His lovingkindness is everlasting.

1 CHRONICLES 16:34 NASB
(EMPHASIS MINE)

Oh give thanks to the Lord, call upon His name;
Make known His deeds among the peoples.

1 CHRONICLES 16:8 NASB 1995

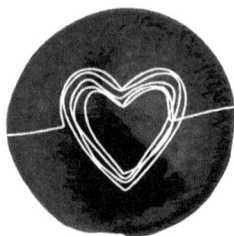

— Father's Heart —

My precious child, you are wired for thankfulness.

When you walk with Me in thankfulness, you become aware of Me in everything. You see Me in nature. You hear Me in relationship.

You experience Me as you were meant to walk—abundant life with Me.

As you choose to give thanks and recognise Me in situations, this is a step of trust and releases faith.

Faith brings powerful uplift.

You are so used to seeing what you lack, yet I have already put much in your hand and have more to bring.

My gifts are waiting in the treasure trove of abundance, waiting for you to choose to trust Me for it. I long to lavish My more upon you.

I have My absolute best for you, My precious child. Don't doubt it for a second. I love you this much.

It is coming and has indeed come.

By abiding in thankfulness, you are aware of and experience Me.

You crush the enemy's plans by living in this way.

Start small and develop this skill.

*You might feel like it isn't doing anything,
but I encourage you—persist.*

*Things around you will begin to change as
a direct result of giving thanks.*

*It will change how you see the very things that
have held you down for so long. Each one an
opportunity to grow, yes, but also to flourish.*

*How much greater is faith when you can walk through
fire and not be burned because of your trust in Me?*

*Will you complain about the heat or thank Me for what I am
bringing you through? Be of good cheer, I am overcoming all
things that oppose My heart in and through you. The things of old
will pale in comparison to that which I have for you, My child.*

Walk through the fire, knowing all the while this will pass.

*Ask Me how I see it, then watch, listen and walk
forward in the provision I have given you for this
moment, giving thanks for what you DO have.*

*You WILL look back upon this time and see
the benefits I have given you in it.*

It is a time of blessing.

Right now, you have things to be thankful for.

*Thankfulness releases. It places hardship in its rightful place.
It places Me in My rightful place—overcoming all! And
remember, I (the One Who overcomes all) am on your side.*

THANKFULNESS

Enter his gates with thanksgiving, and his courts with praise; give thanks to him and praise his name.

PSALM 100:4 NIV

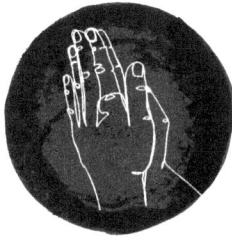

— *Prayer* —

Heavenly Father,

*Help me to walk in thankfulness for
all You have placed around me.*

Thank You for never giving up on me.

*Thank You that You have hope-filled plans
to prosper me for my future.*

*Help me to become so thankful within
that it bubbles up to bless others.*

Thank You, Heavenly Father, for Who You are.

*Thank You for holding nothing back
from me that is for my good.*

*Thank You that I can walk in Your peace at any time of
day or night because of Who and how good You are to me.*

*Thank You for answering every prayer, for
collecting and caring about every tear.*

*Thank You for giving me insight, comfort
and power through Holy Spirit.*

Thank You, precious Father, that NOTHING is wasted in You.

Thank You that I have nothing to fear when I walk with You.

THANKFULNESS

Thank You, Jesus, for overcoming everything for me.

*Thank You, God, that You don't see my
difficulties as reasons to worry.*

Bless You and Your day, precious Father.

Amen.

XXXXX

Be thankful in all circumstances, for this is God's
will for you who belong to Christ Jesus.

1 THESSALONIANS 5:18 NLT

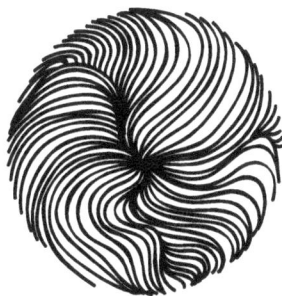

Chapter Fifteen

LAMENT

Out of the depths I cry to you, O Lᴏʀᴅ!
O Lord, hear my voice! Let your ears be attentive
to the voice of my pleas for mercy!

PSALM 130:1-2 ESV

"I will repay you for the years the locusts have eaten —
the great locust and the young locust,
the other locusts and the locust swarm —
my great army that I sent among you.
You will have plenty to eat, until you are full,
and you will praise the name of the LORD your God,
who has worked wonders for you;
never again will my people be shamed.
Then you will know that I am in Israel,
that I am the LORD your God,
and that there is no other;
never again will my people be shamed.

JOEL 2:25-27 NIV

My brother had just been released from prison again…a revolving door of entries and exits over years.

I questioned whether this man before me was out for good this time.

Now a relative stranger, addiction had stolen so much from him and our family.

Although God had healed and redeemed so much in him, I was playing emotional catch-up.

So much emotion. So much history. So much pain. I feel stuck, Lord.

My healing has been in a stall pattern for 20 years.

NOW A RELATIVE STRANGER, ADDICTION HAD STOLEN SO MUCH FROM HIM AND OUR FAMILY.

The mystery of not knowing where he was, if I would still have my brother at all, or whether the early trauma would steal him completely from us—it was a middle death.

No way to move forward, no way to move back to who we once were.

This time feels different, or am I dreaming, Lord?

It had been three years since the God awakening for him when his life came into focus. A miraculous encounter and his whole life changed for the better.

He isn't the same guy I once knew him to be. This is new ground.

How do I move forward, Lord?

IT'S TIME TO
LAMENT, MY
CHILD.

How do I embrace the man before me with so much history behind us? So much has been stolen.

I was a mess of anger and grief—which wrestled with hope and delight as I saw his joy.

It's time to lament, My child.

No need to fear or try and work it all out alone; I am here. It's time to talk about it all.

Lament? Images of sackcloth and waves of tears came to mind.

Lamenting meant "tearing your clothes, covering yourself in ashes, crying and uncomfortable big feelings," doesn't it?

I don't want to be sad; I don't want to spend the week crying. How will this impact my family? What if I start crying and can't stop?

Don't overthink it. It'll be better than you imagine. Trust Me.

I'll show you how to begin.

How long will this time of lament last, Lord?

Seven days.

What will I need?

Your art book and some stationery. Each day I will give you a lament activation. Spend some time with Me, then go on with your day.

Where do I start?

Today I want you to write down all that comes to you. You don't have to accommodate anyone else's feelings here. This is just between You and me. Tell Me all that has happened…all that has hurt you.

I began writing it all down.

It felt strange to write not considering others at all. I could be wholly real.

Don't hold anything back, My beloved.

The invitation had been given, and like a plug being pulled from the clawfoot bathtub filled with my tears, 20 years of pain came pouring out. The more I shared with God, the emptier my bath became.

I poured out the losses and injustices, the disappointments, violations, and anger. I pulled off my filters, my "good-girl" language and held nothing back.

I FELT HIS ARMS
ENFOLD ME AS
I GAVE HIM MY
UNCENSORED PAIN.

A raw, gaping wound finally exposed and brought out into the light.

I felt His arms enfold me as I gave Him my uncensored pain.

Occasional pangs of guilt zipped in.

Years of accommodating others had conditioned me to push my own feelings way down deep, but this was not today's experience.

Today was about my pain alone.

LAMENT

I had to fight to keep it about me. My merciful and loving heart naturally justified and explained away actions, giving grace to all. I wanted to leap ahead to the end result. But the human part of me wanted to, needed to, be heard today, and the lament process was essential to my wholeness.

Keep unloading, My precious one. Don't hold back. This is about your experience of what happened, not anyone else's. Your experience is important and valid.

I pondered my inner tub…the bulk of it was gone. I'd shared all I could think to say. I could see the ring of residue which showed me the depths that had been shared today. The waterline had dropped significantly.

DAY 2.

Today I want you to pour out your heart about how this has impacted your childhood family.

This was a key day as my family had each tried to process and navigate it as best we could. Not wanting to burden one another with what was going on in their own experience of it, but each of us struggling.

I cried out to God with further pain on this day and more emptied from the tub.

Freer and freer it felt.

DAY 3.

Today I want you to tell Me about how this has impacted you, Craig and the children — your grown-up family. How has it impacted you as a family?

"O our God, will you not execute judgment on them? For we
are powerless against this great horde that is coming against
us. We do not know what to do, but our eyes are on you."

2 CHRONICLES 20:12 ESV

Lord, I grieve for family dinners…the loss of normality…the fact that my children have missed out on time together.

Occasional tears welled up, but as I shared with God and asked the tough questions. He responded and eased my pain. Leaving me with a beautiful promise of restoration.

DAY 4.

Today I want you to create a timeline of emotion. Track the primary emotions you've felt over the years.

So I did.

Shock, anger, broken trust, pain, frustration, disappointment, a pessimist's ultimate bucket list. I felt strange putting these empty, but truthful, feelings on paper. As I glanced over the lengthy patterns of emotions and cycles, my heart felt great sadness.

What a waste!

There's nothing good; no one wins here. It's just brokenness from start to finish.

That's true; it is.

No pressure to put a silver lining on it.

It was rare to be heard, without advice, judgment and the pressure to move past something.

This is healing.

I relished the time of being with the only One Who knew, saw it all and was safe enough to hear it all.

Thank You, Father. This feels amazing. What now, Lord?

Now, I want you to go through each emotion, and ask Who I was being for you at this time? I want you to write from My perspective.

My heart leaped at this idea.

How redemptive!

Asking, "Who were you here at this time for me, God?"

Plotting His heart amid it all, I saw the patterns of hope, truth, tenderness and of love. He had been there at every turn, and in every pit.

This too is healing.

DAY 5.

Today I want you to write how this has been for your brother. Write it from what you know of his journey.

Pause.

Oh, Lord.

Putting pen to paper in my journal, the very act of writing became a place where compassion was reignited.

Compassion, which had been ever-present throughout the "tough years"—even when it made no sense.

How many times have I trusted and had that trust dashed?

But time has now proven that it isn't naivety or sticking my head in the sand, but it is God's assurance of well-placed hope.

He is not the same man from all those years ago; he is my prodigal brother restored to us…finally.

And love filled my heart for him, afresh.

Peace.

LAMENT

DAY 6.

I've reached the end of myself. I have nothing left to share.

All has been said, and it feels… finished. What now, Father?

What if you restarted life from today?

What if you accepted him as He is *today*? What if you just loved him as if today was the very beginning?

As I heard these words, my heart swelled with a lightness and freedom, like never before.

Today I want you to write your own psalm. Take all that you've written and pour it into your own psalm.

Nothing was left unexpressed. Getting all that was once on my heart and putting the last few days into a single personal psalm.

It told a story of being heard and nurtured by Him.

Being wholly accepted even with all these disappointments.

Each one, a time where He met with me, with my family, with my brother. Each one, a testimony of His redemptive nature, bringing something good — even in the toughest of times.

Instantly, as I put the final full stop to my psalm, I felt a release of the past — that I'd not experienced in over 20 years.

My tears acknowledged, my heart now free and filled with hope for a brighter future in a healthy relationship with my much-loved brother. Lost…now returned to us in the most magnificent way.

You keep track of all my sorrows. You have collected all my tears in your bottle. You have recorded each one in your book. My enemies will retreat when I call to you for help. This I know: God is on my side!

PSALM 56:8-9 NLT

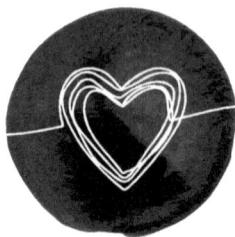

— Father's Heart —

Pour out your heart to Me, My precious one.

I know the griefs of your heart and desire to help you process all that has come against you—all that has sought to wear you down.

Lament, bring Me your woes, cares, worries and pains; nothing is off-limits.

I see the depth of grief and understand.

I care more than you will ever know; let Me tend to those raw and fragile places. Let Me hold you close, as you share from your innermost pain.

Leave nothing out. As you pour it out from heart and head to Me, I will comfort and nurture you, My child.

I hear you. I see you. I care for you. Nothing has gone unnoticed, My child. I have always been with you and am now right here with you.

I know there have been things that you've tried to heal through external measures, counselling, ministry, forgiveness, but there is still residue, consequences of actions, and pain.

Do you feel stuck? There are depths only I can touch.

It's time for us to draw a line in the sand for your pain to be heard, acknowledged and healed through lamenting with Me.

I long to bring you peace.

Doesn't that sound refreshing?

*At times you've have wondered whether you would
ever see the end of this roller coaster — take
heart, there is hope as you share it with Me.*

*There is no rush to resolve or finish up the process, but
for your health, sharing it with Me will help you.*

*You have held it all together, trying to do the "right"
thing. At times you've found it unbearable, wondering
whether you would ever make it through.*

*Please know that bringing your authentic self to me — the person
I already know — brings freedom and healing to your situation.*

*Some things will never be resolved here on
earth, BUT take heart, I have overcome the world.
Peace is available whatever the outcome.*

When you reach the end of yourself, there I am.

*You are not alone, My cherished one. Your pain
is not your own; I am with you in it.*

*Come, let's put aside some time to meet. To share. I
am ready, willing, and able to listen.*

Pour out your raw; leave nothing behind, My darling.

*Then when you've emptied yourself of all that you've
wanted to say, let Me apply balm to the wounds of
life, so that you might heal and have My peace.*

Let Me fill those empty places with gifts straight from My heart.

LAMENT

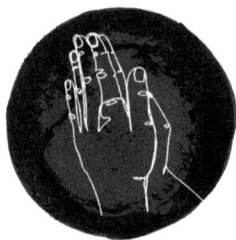

— *Prayer* —

Empowering and compassionate Father,

Thank You that I can share my whole self with You — the raw and the redeemed.

Thank You for being my constant, my safe place, and for holding me close at every turn.

Please show me how to process my circumstances, disappointments, and griefs with You.

Let my ears attune to Your instruction.

Thank You for showing me how I can lament the weighty things of my heart with You.

I trust You to comfort me and tend to my heart, mind and memories.

Lord, I want to fly as free as possible, not held back by anything of the past. Please show me how.

Thank You for giving Jesus to me, Who made a way through even the most disempowering situations. Thank You for being a loving friend, a safe place to land, and the ultimate Redeemer of all things.

In Jesus' powerful name.

Amen.

XXXXX

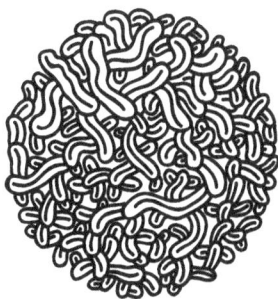

Chapter Sixteen

LEGACY

I have fought the good fight, I have finished
the course, I have kept the faith.

2 TIMOTHY 4:7 NASB

We will not hide them from their children, but tell to the coming generation the glorious deeds of the LORD, and his might, and the wonders that he has done. He established a testimony in Jacob and appointed a law in Israel, which he commanded our fathers to teach to their children, that the next generation might know them, the children yet unborn, and arise and tell them to their children.

PSALM 78:4-6 ESV

called the Institute of Teaching to find out my options. My greatest fear was that I wouldn't be able to remain registered. My four years of study and years of teaching experience would be lost and mean nothing anymore.

The other looming fear was for my identity: *If I am not a teacher, then who am I?*

"If you don't complete one hundred hours of professional development before the end of the year, and weeks of teaching days, then you'll have to redo your entire course. You won't be able to be a registered teacher anymore," the voice on the other end of the line confirmed my worst fears.

This young man with his cool, robotic responses, dashed my hopes in seconds. Even after explaining my situation and having it referred to a superior, the same resolution was given.

Unless you meet our requirements, you'll never teach again, unless you repeat your whole university degree.

My heart dropped into my stomach, and there it remained. Sinking into our couch cushions, I curled up in the fetal position and cried and cried and cried.

There was no accommodating my health, no wiggle room, and therefore no hope for me. It was September and what he had shared was physically impossible for me to complete.

My old life, my only profession, my identity through it—was gone. And I had no idea what was next.

I spent the next week grieving. Tissue box after tissue box was used up. Spontaneous, combustible flows kept coming from my eyes; anything would trigger it. These "attacks" of tears spaced out over time and eventually became less frequent.

> MY OLD LIFE, MY ONLY PROFESSION, MY IDENTITY THROUGH IT — WAS GONE. AND I HAD NO IDEA WHAT WAS NEXT.

I have no idea what's next…but at least I'm not bawling my eyes out anymore.

Looking around at my present day I wondered.

Is this it?

Will I be content for this to be it?

What if this is IT?

Lord, what now? Surely there's more for me…I hope there's something to look forward to. I can't imagine doing anything other than teaching. What next? I don't want to settle for something that isn't right.

One morning a few months later as I journaled with God, I felt a line drop into my heart.

What if you gave it all to Me?

What if you let it all go? Are you willing to allow Me to give you good plans, trusting that I know you best?

I pondered this idea and as I did, I felt internal peace grow at the thought of it.

What if I wasn't a teacher anymore? What if I signed up for God's label for me, rather than my own? What if there's more?!

To support these newfound ponderings, I began seeing the same verse, everywhere.

Jeremiah 29:11 (NIV), "For I know the plans I have for you," declares the LORD, "plans to prosper you and not to harm you, plans to give you hope and a future."

WHAT IF YOU GAVE IT ALL TO ME?

He had given me this promise verse when my health began to go astray. A few weeks after the crash, when everything was falling apart, He gave me this verse and encouraged me.

Hold on. I have good things to come. This isn't the end for you.

He shared that this was My personal promise from Him.

Although physically I was in a no man's land…the "in-between time."

In this period of new mystery and uncertainty, He was present and cared.

Like the perfect coffee and its delicious aroma, anticipation brewed and released a sweet scent into my day.

You have a future and a hope, Karen, that doesn't depend upon your past, your health or anything external. It requires no striving, pushing, or pulling but starts with our taking one step at a time. Before long, you'll find that we've come so far and accomplished great things together. Doesn't that sound appealing? Come let's walk a while, and I will tell you things you could only dare to dream about.

Oh, Lord, that sounds beautiful! Thank You.

Ask Me how I see your future, beloved.

As if frozen in this moment, I stopped still in my thoughts. For some reason, His last comment shocked me.

I began to ask myself some genuine questions.

Do I want to know?

What if I don't like how or what He says?

What if it requires more from me than I've got capacity for?

How will I respond if I don't want what He's offering?

What if...what if....what if....

The thoughts came thick and fast, so I chose not to ask that day.

LIKE THE PERFECT COFFEE AND ITS DELICIOUS AROMA, ANTICIPATION BREWED AND RELEASED A SWEET SCENT INTO MY DAY.

I waited. I wanted to be certain that I was ready to hear His response.

He was patient. He didn't push or shove. He didn't force His will upon mine. He let me come to Him in my own sweet time.

That week, I jostled and wrestled, wrote lists of pros and cons independently of Him as if He couldn't hear my thoughts and musings, fears and failings. It makes me laugh to think about it now, but at the time, it was intense.

I needed to come to a place of peace.

By the end of the week, I found myself yearning for Father's conversation. I wanted to discuss this with Him; He had always been the One I could come to when I had problems to unravel.

I had come to peace about these, but it had taken a lot longer than if I had journeyed it with Him instead. My reasoning was simple. If all the things He had revealed about Himself through this health hardship could be applied now, this is what I knew to be true:

He is always good.

He is for me — not against me.

His nature and personality reveal that I am safe.

I never need to fear what He has to say to me.

I can worry about the what ifs or dive into the actualities.

He is trustworthy. I can trust Him.

And that's what I did.

That same day, I sat down, pen in hand, and journaled three simple words.

"I — am — ready," drawing in a deep breath of nervous anticipation.

"How do You see my future, Father?"

Tentatively and in a whisper I added, "What will life be like if I choose to let go of my life as a classroom teacher?"

I felt His gentle smile on how and what I'd asked. I sensed His enjoyment at finally being able to share it with me.

What if the thing I have for your future gave you *ultimate peace?*

What if it was full of adventure?

What if it was a lot of fun?

What if it brought a complete sense of satisfaction to you?

What if I enabled you to help other people in meaningful ways?

What if it blessed you, your family, and others?

Would you still want to return to teaching?

The list continued with 12 wholesome, wonderful, life-giving elements.

I didn't need a second to reply.

This list. This dream list. My spirit leapt and squealed in delight at the thought that life could hold all these elements.

My reply was a clear and definite no! I don't want to return to teaching if this is what life is like without it.

OH, LORD, THANK YOU, THANK YOU, THANK YOU! I WOULD LOVE LIFE TO BE LIKE THIS!

"God, You can have it!"

Happy to let go of the old, especially when the new met so many of my inner desires and even articulated some I hadn't realised I wanted. I felt like a kid in a candy store as He shared His list.

Oh, Lord, thank You, thank You, thank You! I would LOVE life to be like this!

God's peace poured upon me about my future and what was to come. I dreamed about life and what it might be like to live like this. His list was stunning and wonderful. I returned to this list time and time again. Whenever I felt uneasy about the future, I came back to what He had told me.

Sometime later, I randomly woke up with the idea to contact the Institute of Teaching. I hadn't thought about it in a long time, but I felt a sense of urgency to make the call.

I explained my situation in detail. I told them what the previous man had told me, about my health and about uncertainty that I would ever return to teaching.

I was still peaceful and excited about what God had shared with me but felt it was important to call anyway.

The gentle-hearted lady on the end of the line listened intently. She understood my predicament and showed great compassion and understanding. She then proceeded to tell me I was able to keep my registration for as long as I wanted.

"When you are ready to return," she said, "all you need is ten days of teaching experience, pay the registration fee, and you are back in."

This is incredible news!

I had given up teaching, and He had given it right back to me — if I wanted it.

He had redeemed what had been a grievous situation to my heart.

I found myself sitting in bed, bawling my eyes out-again. Craig and the children came in, worried that something had happened. I told them the story and hugged them so tightly, so joyful that God had restored to me that which was stolen.

I was completely elated!

AFTERWORD

Upon reflection, now years after this event, I can see the very things He promised me all those years ago—have now come to fruition. The elements He shared with me as a future promise—are now a present-day reality.

A deeper, more fulfilling legacy is left by choosing to partner with Him in His story for, me than choosing to live in isolation without Him, doing my own thing.

God is the Ultimate Redeemer. He knows all, sees all, and understands what needs to happen to bring us to the best place that He has prepared for us in advance.

Why wait? This is His legacy for me and for you. Jump in with Him; you'll never look back again!

To obtain an inheritance which is imperishable and undefiled
and will not fade away, reserved in heaven for you.

1 PETER 1:4 NASB

Therefore since we have a great cloud of witnesses surrounding us, let us also lay aside every encumbrance and the sin which so easily entangles us, and let us run with endurance the race that is set before us.

HEBREWS 12:1 BSB

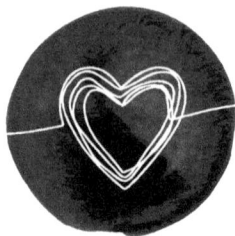

— Father's Heart —

My Word says it time and time again. I redeem broken things and situations because of My love and because of Who I am.

Your circumstances, your hardship, your pains, your thorns — these are what My Son died for.

They are the reason He came; it was for you. He died on the cross for you, but He didn't stay there. If He had, there would be little to no hope. What happened afterward proves that what you have been through and are going through cannot hold you down anymore.

Jesus has risen — from the grave, from sin, from death — He has risen!

He sits by My right side, interceding on your behalf, having overcome the very thing that sought to defeat Him.

Even death, that you sometimes believe is the very worst of things, couldn't keep Him down. He crushed it. He said that it had no power over Him and obliterated it.

And therefore, the things that look to steal, kill and destroy have no authority or power over you anymore.

You are set free because, through His death and resurrection, My Son took care of it for you.

He put the trauma to death on the cross and redeemed the very thing that looked like it was the end. Only it wasn't the end-not by a long shot.

It was truly the end of the beginning.

Give Me your past, whatever that may hold, and I will heal your hurts.

Give Me your present; I will show you the next steps to walking closer with Me, and all the benefits that come with that. I have a legacy for you and for those who follow you, precious one.

Your life is destined to leave its mark upon the world in a most beautiful way.

Give Me your future, and I will display My love for you through the full redemption of what I have done in and through you.

Your story and Mine entwined producing the best of fruit. My legacy given to you through My beloved Son, Jesus.

A day will come when you will look back and realise how much I was at work throughout this situation.

Take heart, precious one. You are My beloved, and I have big plans for you, using your past and springing you into a future full of hope and fullness of joy. Come walk with Me, and I will give you rest. Come, let's talk a while, and I will share with you great and mighty things to come in our US story — things that will give you hope and true freedom.

If you have breath, then I have plans for you, sweet child of Mine. Take heart; I am not limited by life's limitations. Your life story has much life in it yet. Let us continue to make beautiful music together through the US story.

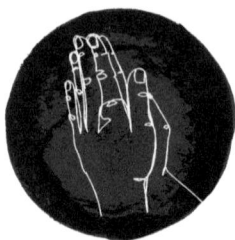

— Prayer —

O Father,

You have proven Yourself to me time and time again.

*I have not always understood Your ways, but You
have opened up the gift of perspective to me.*

I have seen that You were at work all along.

*You have given me delight in walking with You; much of what
used to burden me falls away when I am in Your presence.*

Thank You for the gift of my past.

*Thank You for every experience: positive, traumatic,
upsetting, life-sapping or life-giving moment.*

I trust You when You say that not one of them will be wasted.

Father, please continue to keep my heart soft to the things of You.

*Lord, if and when damage occurs, please heal these
hurts, speak life into dead areas, redeem things that
were meant for harm and use them for good!*

*Father, it is a releasing thing to know You love
to redeem the broken things in our lives.*

Amen.

XXXXX

APPENDIX 1

Below is a brief list of opposite spirit feelings or words that might help to get you started of what can be experienced with God, as He makes exchanges with us.

Hate	Love, affection, treasure, cherished, devotion, kindness, fondness, affection, care, honor
Unforgiveness	Forgiveness, grace, compassion, open arms of love, charity, goodwill, love, mercy, clemency, humanity
Fear	Trust, hope, faith, community, safety, comfort, courage, peace, exchanging heaviness for His light confidence, tenacity, virtue, heart, valiance, bravery
Anxiety/ Worry	Trust, fearlessness, faith, release, support, calm, hope, comfort, joy, assurance, confidence, ease, contentment
Anger	Gentleness, patience, self-control, peace, calm, comfort, joy, delight, tranquillity, stability, unflappability
Hopelessness	Hope, trust, faith, delight, anticipation of good, expectancy of good, healing, optimism, confidence, encouragement, joy, cheer
Depression/ Heaviness	Trust, faith, peace, release, lifting eyes up, contentment, joy, hope, thankfulness, bliss, gladness, happiness, pleasure, contentedness
Rejection	Acceptance, love, warmth, comfort, approval, embrace, support, security, a place of welcome, reception, acknowledgement, received

Isolation/ Loneliness	Community life, never alone, befriended, accepted, accompanied, embraced, togetherness, intimacy, fellowship, company, friended by Jesus
Control	Submission to God and His ways, trusting Him, relinquish, freedom, let go, finding ourselves in a place of enough, liberated, unconstrained, contented
Despair/ Discouragement	God's acceptance, God's truth, joy, peace, building anticipation, encouragement, filled up, hope, supported, comforted, lifted, faith, peace, joyful
Guilt/Shame	Jesus having died on the cross with all our sin, forgiven, free, virtuous, honoured, refreshed, light, acquitted, released, restored dignity, respected
Affliction/ Poor health	Perfect health, fullness of the Holy Spirit within, freedom, trust, healthy, carefree, lighter, hopeful, soothed, comforted, healed, tended to, supported, strong, provided for, whole, robust
Pride	Submission to God and His leading, humility, release of control, modest, freedom, thankfulness, grace, innocent, peace, secure in His ability
Insecurity	Trust, security, strength, fearlessness, stable, safe assurance, courage, protection, firm, assured, unafraid, released, free
Tempted	Strength, trust, truth, submission to God, released, courage, assured, secure, wisdom

Every night the dreams had become almost like clockwork — dream after dream after dream.

My whole world was being turned upside down, or right side up.

"Father, whether or not I sleep, You can have my night-time. You've got the next eight or so hours of uninterrupted time. You have my full attention. Please protect me from any influences outside of You and Your will. Use this time to draw my heart closer to Yours, precious Father. In Jesus' name, amen."

Jesus, sleep is evading me. Can You take me on one of Your adventures?

Often within seconds, I would find a picture came to mind — an environment, a place, a person's face — always with Jesus smiling there at me. I'd take His hand, and we'd begin. And before I knew it, I was waking up, having had some incredible dreams whilst sleeping.

PRACTICAL/STRATEGIC DREAM ANSWERED

I had felt concerned about a situation at church where our precious deaf sister and brother were without someone to sign the sermon for them. There didn't seem to be an easy solution, and I saw their frustration and isolation. Holy Spirit gave me eyes to see what was going on, and I didn't like it — not one bit.

I went to bed that night subconsciously asking for help with the problem. Quite miraculously, when I woke up, I had dreamt of a solution. He had shown me that using a laptop and a keyboard could communicate the message, when there wasn't an interpreter available. God had given a practical solution. Praise Him!

Following the initial dream encounters with God, I began to take them a little more seriously. He began to use this time together as a blessing to me, as well as to others.

ACTION DREAMS

I once had a dream about a single Mum and her large family. In the dream I rang her and prayed a blessing over her and her children, individually.

I decided that even if it wasn't a direct instruction dream, it couldn't do any harm, so I called up this total stranger and introduced myself.

She was a little wary initially, but unbeknownst to me, she was having a challenging time.

I explained what I sensed God asking me to do and asked for her permission to pray with her for her children.

She agreed, and we spent the next little while together on the phone.

I prayed for her family, and she wept with joy as we blessed her children by name and gave prophetic words of encouragement about each one.

Bringing her God's encouragement was such a delight, and as a side note, be a part of His story for her in a small way.

I learnt through this experience that God loves us to sometimes engage with what He shows us in dreams and run with the ones that reflect His heart for the world. Dreams are powerful!

GOD HAS REDEMPTIVE VERSIONS OF
EVERY DREAM, INCLUDING THE BAD ONES

I once had a nightmarish dream about babies who were drowning. My heart raced, and I felt petrified as I woke having observed this terrible scene. After asking Him about the dream, He revealed that the babies represented new kingdom ideas, and the drowning was not drowning but immersing under water. Water is often symbolic of Holy Spirit. This was a GOOD dream!

HEALING/REASSURING DREAMS

I once had an older friend who was shaken by the dream she had had the previous night. In it, she was sleeping with another man; she felt shame upon waking from the dream, and this dream left her troubled throughout her day.

As I sat with her and listened, I sensed that the man in her dream was Holy Spirit and sleeping with Him represented intimacy with Him.

As I asked her whether this resonated with her, she immediately began to tear up; that very week she had been desiring to be closer to God.

The dream made complete sense to her now, and she was so relieved at the truth God had given her, that He too desired closeness with her, and it was happening.

God's heart is for purity and intimacy; it's sometimes our brokenness or cultural outlook that can twist something that is pure and good from God.

WARNING DREAMS

I have had dreams where I saw something that was about to happen and felt a sense of wariness as I woke. Some of these we have acted upon, and everything has gone smoothly. Others we have not, and the very thing God prepared us for happened, as in the dream. I have learnt that He uses dreams to sometimes warn us or prepare us.

PRACTICAL/PREPARATION DREAMS

Recently I had a practical dream where my husband and daughter were going away on a five-day bike ride. The event was being catered for, and as such, I was concerned in the dream about whether my daughter, who is a plain eater would be able to eat what was provided. The next day I shared this dream with my husband who then sent me the menu via email. Every day was curries and meals that our daughter wouldn't eat. In the dream God had shown me putting tins of salmon and other items in their pack. And this is what we did.

Praise God that He wanted to ensure she had plain, healthy food to eat while away. I have learnt that God cares about the seemingly small things in our lives.

DREAMS FOR OTHERS/STRATEGIC INSIGHTFUL DREAMS

God once gave me a dream for a friend who, unbeknownst to me, was going through some very heavy trials in their business. They had employed a family member who was not behaving honourably, which was putting them in a moral dilemma of epic family proportions. This situation was creating an intense amount of stress for this precious friend.

God gave me a symbolic dream which I shared with her. Thankfully (although it was a mystery to me), it was very clear to them. He encouraged them and clarified some elements of what was going on in their circumstance. He even spoke in language that both she and her husband understood and used symbols that only this couple knew about that I couldn't have known apart from God. I learnt through this dream that God is creative and personal in dreams.

MYSTERY-SOLVING DREAMS

More recently, I woke up having had a wonderfully encouraging dream that healed a broken part of my heart. I had walked with some deep grief about whether my grandfather was with God. I had come to peace that I would never know this side of heaven. In this dream, a young man (my grandfather) showed me what was wrong with my camera. (My actual camera was broken at the time.)

After this night, God gave me clarity without any doubt. I know because of the dream that my grandfather is with my Heavenly Father. I had never actually asked God the question; I was concerned that I wouldn't like the answer, but He knew the question was deep in my heart of hearts.

The entire morning after, I sang praises to God, that He had healed some deep hurts and sealed answers to old mysteries. Thanks to God Who knows what we need and when we need it. I learnt through this dream that God loves to give us answers to questions we haven't even articulated with our mouths. And to make it even better, when I took my camera to the camera shop, the assistant showed me which button I needed to press to fix the issue — the exact one the young man had shown me in the dream.

God loves to meet with us in dreams and bring whatever is needed. Take heart! Everyone dreams, whether we remember them, or not.

If He has put it on your heart to dream with Him, ask, expect and put a journal by your bedside.

I find the most important things often happen right as I drop off to sleep and shortly before I wake. He will often repeat really, really important information, e.g., the same word or picture will show up again and again.

He often uses familiar people, places, and things so that they will stay in the place we can remember. Sometimes those people, places and things represent something entirely different.

When we have dreams, it's fun to talk to God about them, asking Him to reveal their meaning.

"I am the branches; you are the leaf.

Come, connect to My life-giving branches once again.

Let Me pour life back into you.

Let Me restore your color.

Let Me hold you once again.

My arms are open wide and ready to
embrace your battle-weary form.

In the natural, a young leaf is green, full of hope and
life. The elements seem to come relentlessly.
Eventually, the wind, rain, and storms wear it down,
and the now colorless frail leaf falls from the tree lifeless.

But with Me, this isn't the end, but the beginning.

I am counter-cultural and counter-intuitive.

Where you may feel that your situation
has sucked the best years from you,

That all is hopeless.

That there is no coming back from this place of upheaval,

Take heart with Me. This is not the case!

You come to Me, dry, brittle, worn-out and weary,
and I pour Myself into those desert places.

As I hold you, I pour My life into you.

I apply balm to your well-trodden, wilderness areas.

I restore your color.

I give you back life and bright eyes.

I lead you to green places of flourish.

Where the world saps the life from you,
I give you life and life to the full.

Take heart, My precious one, I am not limited by what you
see or feel—there is HOPE and much future to be had.

You can come back from this and thrive with Me.

My beloved, this isn't the end of you, but the
beginning of something new in you as you
allow Me to embrace you once again."

ENCOURAGEMENT FOR THOSE ON A

Spiritual Journey

WHO WANT TO CONNECT WITH GOD FOR THEMSELVES

First, welcome; thank you for picking up my book.

You could have looked at countless books; I'm thankful that you landed here. Whatever led you here, I am confident that it's no mistake. This page is just for you if you are on a spiritual journey and want to know more about and encounter God for yourself.

No doubt, God has some encouragement for you—yes, even in your own challenging time. He loves all people, and the good news is that it includes us both. You've read some of my experiences with Him through this book, and no doubt you'll have your own to share as well.

If we met in everyday life, we'd probably be sitting down with a cuppa (cup of tea/coffee) and having a good conversation about life, faith, and whatever else came up.

We'd possibly share about our tough seasons and our challenges, but also the incredible things—those unexplainable moments which can only come from something outside of ourselves—that have happened along the way. These kinds of encounters are exciting to hear and to talk about with one another.

I'd be celebrating your unique God design and cheering you on in your journey. I love nothing better than doing this with whoever God brings along my path.

I know that you'd leave having been encouraged by Him, and I'd feel blessed for having met you. Although I appreciate your being here and taking a bold step forward in faith and exploration, this obviously isn't our meeting in person, which got me to thinking, *How does this happen through the pages of a book? How do I encourage someone I might never meet or talk with? What advice would I give to those who want to know God for themselves?*

So I began asking God for some advice. What steps do I take that have helped me connect with Him best? He answered me through a dream, and I wrote down the five steps He showed me.

1. BEGIN.

When I say *begin*, I mean start asking God to speak in a way that you understand.

Start talking to Him about everything. If you have questions, ask them.

Nothing is off-limits when it comes to talking to God.

Talking to God can be implemented through speaking verbally, journaling, or thinking with Him. Our "hows" do not limit Him, He is more interested in connecting rather than how you choose to connect with Him. He wants to be heard as much as you want to hear Him.

2. FOSTER AN AWARENESS OF HIM.

Keep watch, wait and take note of what He is saying, showing you, and how you sense He is communicating with you in the everyday.

Some of the ways He speaks are found in this book series, but there are soooooo many more. Chances are, He has already been talking to you. You might not have recognized that God's voice doesn't necessarily sound like a Morgan Freeman voiceover, mystical, loud, or booming.

His voice can be the voice you hear in the quiet—the gentle prompting. Or when you feel your heart respond to something, this can be His Spirit leading you.

If you've ever felt or experienced love, joy, peace, kindness, patience, goodness, hope, or any other life-giving aspect, this IS God speaking. Without Him, these virtues would not exist.

Has something drawn your eye? Has something out of the ordinary happened? God is often in these too.

Nothing is off-limits when it comes to how God can communicate with you. Take note of those times when you are tended to, encouraged, or lifted. These kinds of help bear the heart of God.

Once you start noticing Him and taking note of His voice, you'll see He is always present and speaking with you.

3. START READING.

Get yourself a Bible or use a bible app. Plenty of options are available; I have found YouVersion is a great resource.

Start with the book of Mark. It talks about the life of Jesus, and none of this means anything without Jesus.

When exploring online, a plethora of options are available. How do we navigate this with wisdom? I find it's healthy to ask questions about anything I read:

- Is what I'm reading reflecting Jesus' heart and nature?

- Is it supported by the teachings of the Bible?

- Does it draw me closer to God and a healthy relationship with Him?

If it does all these things, then you are off to a good start.

4. FIND YOUR KIND OF PEOPLE.

We all need one another, so look out for and connect with a healthy local church or Christian community where we can grow together and encourage one another.

Ask God to show you where to start.

Understand that most churches differ in terms of worship styles and some beliefs. It's good to find one which fits how God has designed you to connect with Him.

5. CHECK OUT THE ALPHA WEBSITE.

This site (alpha.org.au) is a safe place to ask all those nagging questions and to wrestle with the significant issues. It's also an excellent resource for further information about Jesus and becoming a Christian.

God doesn't require you to work or strive to be loved by Him. He doesn't require you to be good enough to have a relationship with Him. He naturally wants to reveal Himself to those who want to get to know Him.

He's incredibly personal and wholly relational, and best of all, whether you know Him, He loves you 100 percent. Nothing you could do will ever change this unconditional love of His. It's great news!

I will be praying that your spiritual journey will be the best adventure of your life.

However you choose to take the next step, know that He is closer than you think, cares about you and all that you are going through, and has ways for you to flourish despite circumstances.

I hope you will thoroughly enjoy getting to know Father God in the way He has planned for you. I know it'll bless your life; I know this because I've lived the truth of it for decades. Woah, that makes me feel really old. Lol! But it's true!

God bless you, precious one; I'll be praying for you.

xxxxx

Thankfest

I couldn't finish my final book in the 'Be Held by Him' series, without a quick thankfest!

Writer's life is never done alone, (even though it can feel like it at times.) There are a plethora of supporters, resourcers, helpers, and prayer warriors who have gone into bat for me over the past decade—that I want to acknowledge and thank.

PERSONAL THANKFEST

To my supernatural Father, words cannot hope to express my gratefulness to You. You've not left me for a second. You've revealed so much of Yourself to me in this time; it's made the whole thing worthwhile. The richness that comes in getting to know You personally is beyond what I could have hoped for in my life.

You've amazed me. You've inspired me. You've been everything You've promised You'd be, and more. Life is worth living when it's lived with You in my heart. I'm looking forward to diving into the more of You over the coming decades and beyond. They say it takes a village to raise a child; well, You've given me my village in this time, and I am forever grateful for them today.

To my precious hubby Craig.

How do I honor someone who has been my best friend for all these years? We promised to remain with one another through sickness and health, but neither of us could have conceived that this might be our path. This past decade you've loved and cared for us all. You've tended to me when I needed help. Whether it be a hydralyte, a hot water bottle, or a hug, your kindness is something that I will always be thankful for. I know it's been hard watching from the side and being unable to fix it, but thank you for sticking by me—thank you for not giving up. Thank you for growing in this with me; I love who we are now. And I can honestly say I'm unsure we would be where we are, without having walked this hard, hard road. Thank you for being the best hubby a girl could pray for and the best dad I could ever want for our kids. I love you, honey, and am looking forward to what God has in store for us over the coming decades and beyond.

To our kids, Cameron, Hannah, and Ryan, I love you. I love you. I love you. On one level, I want to say, I'm sorry. I'm sorry that your childhoods have not been what others have walked. I'm sorry you've had a Mum who didn't always have the energy, patience, transportation or capacity other Mums did; I know that it has been difficult for you sometimes…and for those times, I am sorry. But I don't wish it was different; there are no regrets.

This experience has also given us something others don't get much of. Time. Time together. An awareness of God's tangible presence in our home and lives. It's brought us closer together. It's united us in many ways. It's developed characteristics in you which have helped equipped you for life— albeit a little earlier than I would've naturally planned, but you know how to feed yourselves, do the laundry, and very rarely complain of being bored. You know how to be by yourselves and to be content in that. You have lived out this faith walk with me, and seen, experienced God's hand in so many life challenges. My hope is that this is something you draw from and learn from in your adult lives. It's a rare and precious fringe benefit of this season. One which I'm sure will help in your own difficult times of life. I pray that God will turn your hard times for good as well.

Cam, your gentle, quiet, steady heart and head, have been gifts to me in this time. Your hugs are healing; I've always known that, but in this season, I've experienced it. I love your faith, your commitment, your compassion, your inherent loyalty, your sense of humor is an absolute cracker. The endless watchfests of The Crown, Father Brown, Agatha Cristie classics, I so enjoy spending time with you. I admire and find myself smiling as I see your heart for all things books and media. I love that you prioritise voluntary work and serving others. I love that you are following your dreams, and I look forward to continuing to cheer you on, my son, my friend.

Hanny, your joy and boundless tiggerness, your sweet heart in this season have been so appreciated, darlin'. Whether you've made an egg sandwich or brought me a hydralytye, a blanket, or a hug, your nurturing and kind heart is something I am so grateful for. Your sense of fun and natural propensity for joy has brought laughter to my heart, when all I felt like doing was cry. You teach me so much. I could not have wanted a better daughter. I love your willingness to run groups that bless others, invest in others through your encouraging words—I can see how God is partnering with you day by day. I love that you are honorable, teachable, fiercely loyal. Like a magnet, you draw others to the heart of God and to life. It's beautiful to watch. God bless you, precious daughter and friend.

Ryan, your creativity, kindness, sensitivity in this season have been so priceless. You've made me precious cards and creations which have brought tears to my eyes. You've cuddled up on the couch and been content to pass the time with me. I love that you ask questions and want to know. I love how God has given you insight into things others struggle to understand. I love that you have ideas — loads of ideas, and no doubt, God will partner with you to see many of these come to fruition. I love and appreciate your honesty, even when it's hard. This is the making of a true and honorable man! I love watching you grow and mature, I admire how you fast and pray. My Mumma heart smiles big when you choose to draw near to Jesus. I love that you do hard things — things that make you uncomfortable just because you know that's what's right for you. Well done, precious sonno and friend.

You have all inspired me and brought joy to me by being yourselves. It gives me great pleasure to see you grow and have fun along the way. I love how we engage as a family and individually. I love that Dad and I get to cheer you on for the rest of our lives in whatever you do and wherever God leads you. Keep close to Him, darlings, and you'll never lack hope, faith, or love.

To my precious family, you have carried me when it mattered most. You've prayed. You've brought meals and ferried kids everywhere. You've probably shed tears I will never know anything about. Please understand that these unseen acts have brought much fruit. This book is just one part of what you've enabled me to do with God. Without you, life would be far less. I am thankful for you all, for your lives, for your kindness to me, to us, especially in this time. Thank you for those late-night conversations and the hugs (and everything else that is listed in the friend section too. Lol). I bless you and thank you for all that you've done, but most importantly, I value all that you are as people. I would choose you even if you weren't my family. XXXXX

To those special friends (you know who you are): the prayers, the meals, the car trips, the help, the cleaning, the acts of service and love, the pallets of tissues, the hugs, the messages, cards, sms' of hope, the smiles, the words of encouragement, and thoughts—thank you for these and so much more. Thank you for holding up a mirror to my face when I needed to see how God saw things. Thank you for lifting me up physically, emotionally, spiritually when everything of the old me physically fell apart. Thank you for sticking by me. Thank you for never giving up— for being real with me and allowing me safe spaces to download. Although you didn't live in my body, you saw enough to know that things were pretty dire at times. You spoke hope and life over me in loving embrace. You showed me what a village experience is like and left me wanting this to be the norm for everyone. Saying you were Jesus with skin on feels cliché, but it's true. I am thankful for you and pray often for God's blessing in your lives. I love and appreciate you, not because of what you do for me, but who you are. *XXXX*

To my God-given medical/health village (you know who you are): your depth of heart, knowledge, and kingdom insight has me upright and enjoying life to the fullest possible extent. You have helped this dream of healthy living become more of a reality. You've tended to my system, spoken hope, followed strings to come to revelations that have given greater freedoms and healing. I cannot tell you how much I love you and am grateful for your sacrifices along the way. It's no easy path to walk differently from others, but this difference has made a difference for me. You are out-of-the-box thinkers, believers, and doers. Those truths have made this out-of-the-box girl with out-of-the-box body systems a LOT healthier and happier because of your unique hearts and skills. When mainstream medicals had no idea, you did. You walk closely with God, and I thank Him for you often and bless you in my prayers.

Thank you for going the extra mile for me — thank you for answering frantic calls, for genuinely caring, for everything you've done to help. You've blessed my physical body, my emotional, mental, and spiritual life exponentially. God bless you with decades more of adventuring with Him, with one another, discovering all that Holy Spirit has available to His children. Sending you all my love. *XXXX*

To my church pastors, leaders, and family, you barely knew me when this all began. You gave me water to drink when my soul was parched. You visited, prayed for, and with me; you tended to me on more occasions than I can count. These books reflect many of the times you invested in me. Thank you. Thank you. Thank you. You gave language to the things I was experiencing with God; you taught me so much about Holy Spirit. I love being a part of Peninsula City Church; it has become an extension of my home because of the precious people who attend. You've given me more than I could hope to repay, but I thank God for you and hope, in some form, you will be blessed as a result of your investment in me in this season. I love you all. XXXXX

To my connect groups and prayer friends,

You know just how much this series has been a journey of ups and downs. Thankyou for supporting me, thankyou for praying for these books. Thankyou for putting up with my ranting when things weren't going smoothly, I hope that you've enjoyed watching from the sidelines—just how God has redeemed the LOT! I certainly have from within it.

Thankyou for being an integral part of my support network, and reciprocal friendship circles. I have needed you for so long, and when you arrived—my heart flew! I thoroughly enjoy doing life with you all. I love celebrating your wins, praying for one another, and being there for you when things aren't all sunshine and rainbows.

You are my church family and I love you.

Thankyou also, for commissioning me in this calling to write—your vision of my this writing life, has often been bigger than I have felt myself—but the God mirror you share with me has drawn me up—and these books are just a small offering of the fruit from your love investments. Your continual encouragement and gentle words of hope, have helped exponentially, to keep me pressing in—until God revealed the next step. Thankyou for your faithfulness, Sue, Julie, Lizzy, Katharine, Anne, Elizabeth, Lara, Lisa, Emma and of course my original Wendy's connect group chicky babes.

A girl couldn't ask for better friends and prayer warriors.

Love you sooooo much.
XXXXX

WRITER'S LIFE THANKFEST

I was given the gift of walking alongside a couple of writer friends, especially closely in the first series, but both women are power-houses for God.

Jane Berry (janeberryauthor.com), and Beth Kennedy (VerveMin-istries.com).

I am acutely aware, and thankful for the impact you have both played in my book journey. Your consistent encouragement, advice, wisdom, prayers, and words of prophecy have helped me at key times in recent years. I'm not sure I would have gotten through this without you.

Although we haven't formally met as a writing group since lock-down, those seeds planted in the early years, have gone on to help produce this book series. God brought us along one another's paths at just the right time!

And now I have the honor of watching and cheering, as God con-tinually works powerfully through you both.

Beth, as you zoom ahead with Him, speaking nationally and inter-nationally, your heart is all about the importance of stopping for the one—I LOVE this about you.

You are by far, the most honoring person I have ever met—and you've inspired me greatly in my faith walk, personal life and in the way I celebrate and lift others—and honor them. If only the world would walk in a way that celebrates, rather than competes with one another—wouldn't it be a wonderful world to live in! You in your own way, make this happen, and inspire others to walk the same way. I know for me it has been life changing.

We share a passion for the one, and for hearing God's voice. I love your style, courage, heart and all that God is leading you into. You've give up much, and I am trusting that God will bless you greatly for it!

I know that anyone who is wise and blessed enough to check out your God stories, soaking sessions and prophetic activations and teaching, will be forever changed and blessed beyond belief—just as I have been. www.VerveMinistries.com

Jane, we have been friends for decades now, but you never cease to amaze me. Your willingness to step in and help others, your dedication and commitment to all things family and marriage. You are a true servant heart and bless many who come along your path.

Jane your honest prayers and those 'emergency' downloads have been such a gift to me in this season, and in life. I appreciate your generosity in praying with me at times where the weirdest things have happened, and without skipping a beat, you offer to pray. Thankyou for being unshakable with Him!

I love the way your children get to shine, as you help them navigate life and become all that God has created them to be. This fresh new season where you and Gary are starting a podcast on hearing the voice of God—will be so empowering. I am so looking forward to listening in and learning more. I trust that it will be world changing as you move into fresh new seasons.

To my precious and God-given graphic designer Abigail: how God brought you across my path is nothing short of miraculous! As I spoke to you about my book, I sensed Holy Spirit saying, "Give her free rein." You intuitively understood my heart and desire for my readers; you created something that makes these words shine. I'm thrilled with you and what you've created with Him! Thank you for taking the time to invest in us.

To my brilliant Editor Linda, wow! Linda, you've been such a gift to me and this project. I am so thankful to God for how He brought you miraculously into my life. An initial recommendation for Affordable Christian Editing, a stunning hearted ministry and business.

Publishing can be expensive and I wanted to steward it well, considering I needed to do six books, instead of the usual one at a time. God knew. The moment I saw your photo on the website, I felt I knew you. And then to have you be the one who responded with an offer to edit, well, it was no surprise. I LOVED that you didn't change my voice. You edited with such professionalism and warmth. You engaged with the subject matter and gave me fabulous and encouraging feedback. Only God can have known how the content would speak to you and encourage you. Only He could have known that we were to have eventually met. I honor you darlin, for your investment in this book baby series, in my process and in my life. I love your spunk, passion, diligence and authenticity. God bless you and yours greatly for your goodness and generosity. XXXXX

To the precious Stacey, well, what a process we've been on Stacey. Only God can have worked it all out. The initial recommendation only to realise that the subject matter of the book was something your were all too familiar with. You have been an answer to prayer on so many levels. It was a delight to meet you and get to speak to someone who has walked a similar journey. Not to mention the incredible way God used the book to bring a little light during a particularly tough season for you and your family. Only God can bring that about. I'm so thankful for your honorable spirit. I applaud the amazing map you've created, with very little input from me. I had no idea what to expect and it's so much better than anything I could ever have imagined. I know it wasn't the easiest thing to plot all the chapter subjects, but you've done it, and done it beautifully. God bless you precious daughter of His. God bless your Mumma heart and your creativity with a line straight from heaven. XXXXX

To my fantastic book cover designer and formatter Steve, you were sooooo patient with the process. Like a dependable ship unwavering in focus and skill. You helped me navigate the waters of an area I knew nothing about. Another US import, you worked with the

Aussie girl through late afternoon zooms having the patience of a saint. Again I was led to employ your services, through many God confirmations. I couldn't be happier with what you've produced and I LOVE how you've worked the interior and exterior of the book so professionally. I would highly recommend you to anyone looking for a faith fella, who is reliable, communicative and prompt. Steve, these qualities and more are what set you apart from the rest. Thankyou, thankyou, thankyou!

To my writers groups online, Flourish Writers and the fabulous Mindy and Jenny!

Mindy our coaching session have helped me more than I could hope to articulate in a single paragraph. Thankyou for you faithfulness, love and kindness to me. Thankyou for holding my hand and my heart gently and your helpt shine a light onto the next step.

To Chad Allen & Jodie from the Bookcamp community—I am so grateful for your cheerleading, pick me ups, solid teaching and providing a safe place for me—a home for part of my heart.

It's been a gift to me to have your cutting edge author world insight. Your feedback, constructive suggestions, coaching, mentoring and inspired ways of thriving as an author.

These communities of writers are beyond amazing! I would recommend anyone hoping to write their book, to sign up and connect with your communities—because they are 'that' GOOD. Thankyou for believing in me, and in my message.

Much Love to you all,

Karen
XXXXX

ABOUT THE AUTHOR

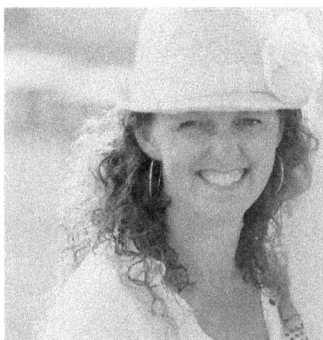

Karen Brough is an Australian wife, mother, writer, and former primary school teacher. She is the author of the *Be Held by Him* series, *Finding God when Life Knocks You Off Your Feet* and is currently working on some children's books with heart (and funny bone)—she is very excited to share updates with her subscribers—**karenbrough.com**

Ten years ago, when hit by a mystery illness, Karen began sharing the encouragements God gave her via her blog.

Her unique voice makes her readers feel understood, inspired, hopeful and encouraged. She spurs others on to connect with Father God for themselves by sharing the adventures she has with Him in everyday life.

Karen has always had a passion for writing and for encouraging others and cannot remember a time without this gift. Her blog has been read and enjoyed both domestically and internationally.

She loves nothing better than to spend time with her husband and three children. In warmer months, you'll often find her body boarding and making sand castles at the beach; or lying by the pool doing crosswords and creating "healthy" gelato for anyone who might drop by.

In cooler weather, she loves jigsaws, rom coms, bubble baths and baking anything warm, comforting and delicious—often hiding vegetables in sweet muffin recipes, much to her children's disgust. (Secretly they love it though.) She is still yet to find the perfect dairy free gelato recipe.

She loves the slower, unhurried pace of life and following this past health-challenge season, desires God's peace above all else.

She loves to laugh, cry and love with her whole heart, and wants to leave this earth a whole lot better than when she came into it. She loves nothing better than to help others see their value and worth, and help them fly to even greater heights in life, love and faith.

Nevertheless, I will bring health and healing to it; I will heal my people and will let them enjoy abundant peace and security.

JEREMIAH 33:6 NIV

CONNECT WITH US

We Love to hear from readers: If you have been impacted by this book, please consider getting in touch with us.

or

Leave a review on Amazon or Goodreads, so others can benefit from your personal experience. (this also helps get the word out about the books)

It takes a village to make the world go round, and you are an important part of our village.

FREE RESOURCES FOR MY READERS:
KARENBROUGH.COM/FREE-RESOURCES/

FACEBOOK: KARENBROUGHAUTHOR

INSTAGRAM: KARENBROUGHAUTHOR
KARENBROUGHKIDS

WEBSITE: KARENBROUGH.COM

Writing can be quite an isolating space, so we LOVE hearing from you.

Has the book impacted your life; your relationship with God?

Do you have a testimony of His goodness in your own hard time?

Or if you have any encouragements, fan art or inspirational creations that might help inspire or affirm others, share and connect with your online village on the "Be Held by Him" Facebook page or email us at **beheldbyhimseries@gmail.com**

GOD BLESS YOU DEARLY, BRAVE ONE.

Precious Reader,

It's with a touch of sadness that I see the end of this series, it has truly been a work of heart, tears, patience, and vulnerability. It has cost me greatly at times, but on the flip side, has also given me so much fruit as well.

I pray it has given you a gift along the way too.

I am looking forward to future writing projects (as prompted by Him), and in the meantime, there is still plenty to share, and to celebrate—and I do this on my website and social media. If you liked these kinds of stories, I blog these regularly at karenbrough.com.

I love hearing from my readers and always try to respond personally to each and every letter.

For those who have already reached out, thankyou for your kind words, your stories that have come about as a result of reading the series. Your testimonies of His fingerprint in your lives have been like honey for my heart—these encourage me greatly!

Let's never give up in being wowed by His goodness in it all.

God bless you and keep you, make His face shine upon you, and give you peace.

God knows we all need help at times and drawing closer to Him is always the best idea!

Much love, Karen
XXXXX

P.S. BONUS: I have created a dedicated resources page on my website, brimming with free resources, blessings, story-behind-the-story clips, and sneak peeks just for you. You can easily access it by visiting the website and clicking on the "Resources" tab.

Moreover, my website friends receive special encouragements, blessings, and plenty of funny memes to lighten the load with each email. If you appreciate being encouraged, blessed, and finding laughter in the lighter side of life, you might have found your people!

Sending much love, Karen

XXXXX

Have you read others in this series?

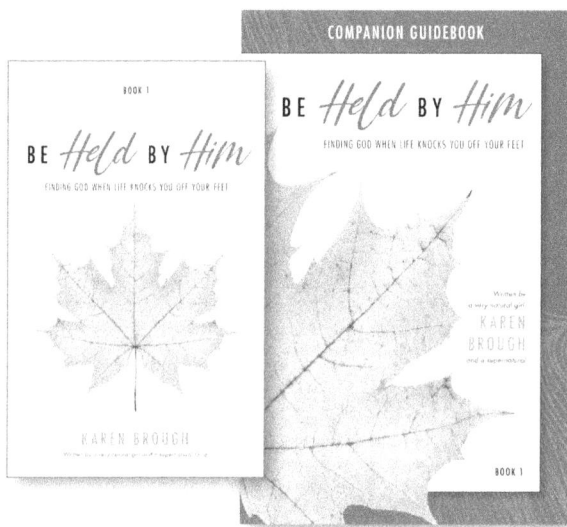

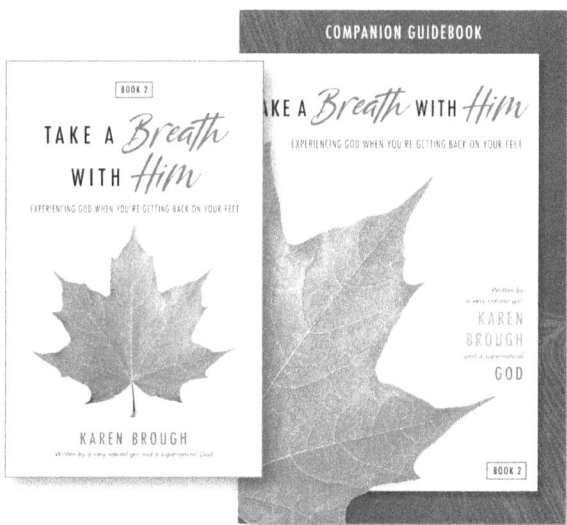

BOOK 1

BE *Held* BY *Him*

FINDING GOD WHEN LIFE KNOCKS YOU OFF YOUR FEET

KAREN BROUGH

COMPANION GUIDEBOOK

BE *Held* BY *Him*

FINDING GOD WHEN LIFE KNOCKS YOU OFF YOUR FEET

KAREN BROUGH

BOOK 1

BOOK 2

TAKE A *Breath* WITH *Him*

EXPERIENCING GOD WHEN YOU'RE GETTING BACK ON YOUR FEET

KAREN BROUGH

COMPANION GUIDEBOOK

TAKE A *Breath* WITH *Him*

EXPERIENCING GOD WHEN YOU'RE GETTING BACK ON YOUR FEET

KAREN BROUGH

GOD

BOOK 2

Karen's latest children's book release:

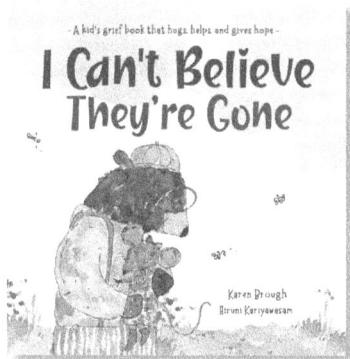

I CAN'T BELIEVE THEY'RE GONE
A Kid's Grief Book that Hugs, Helps and Gives Hope,' now available!

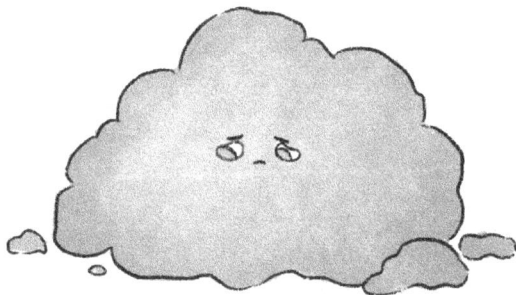

THE LITTLE BLACK CLOUD is on its way!

Subscribe for the news on her latest children's book titles
karenbrough.com

www.ingramcontent.com/pod-product-compliance
Lightning Source LLC
Chambersburg PA
CBHW052010030426

42334CB00029BA/3163